MEDICAL ILLUSTRATION

The **Medical Illustration Source Book** *was created 14 years ago to visually bring medical illustrators and medical art buyers together for their mutual benefit. At that time, there was no other visual resource designed specifically to do this. According to our national surveys, the Source Book has been spectacularly successful in achieving this goal. Art directors, editors, product managers, journal publishers, medical educators, marketing directors and others have repeatedly told us that this book has become an indispensable tool in locating the country's top talent in medical illustration.*

No other source book does a better job nationwide, of serving *your* needs as a medical art buyer. The **Medical Illustration Source Book** brings to you the most pages (almost two hundred) of the nation's top medical art talent. It is a source book that is easy to use. Spiral bound to lie flat on your desk for convenience, it is indexed alphabetically and divided into B&W and color sections. Besides each illustrator's artwork, there is also valuable information on their professional training, education, and areas of special medical expertise.

In these days of budget restraint and potential government oversight, you as a medical art buyer can't afford the risk of wasting time and money on visual communication that might be visually ineffective or scientifically inaccurate. The **Seventh Edition** of the **Medical Illustration Source Book** places at your fingertips access to a vast resource of medical and scientific information through the medical artists represented here. You can take advantage of their extensive training and in-depth knowledge of anatomy, physiology, pathology, surgery, and other medical specialties. You can take advantage of their enormous store of "hands on" medical experience. *You can make your job easier - all for the price of a phone call.*

S0-AZS-162

Cover Art By:
The Studio of Paul Peck, Ph.D.:
 Paul Peck, Ph.D. (1908-1982)
 Lou Bory
 Ray Srugis
 José Alemany

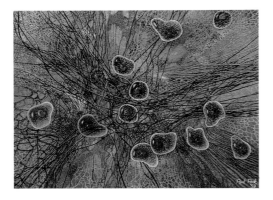

Title:
The Reticuloendothelial System.
This art is one of a series of twelve paintings from the body of work entitled "The Poetry of the Body." The paintings are owned and on display at the U.S. Human Health Headquarters of Merck & Co., Inc.

Meduim:
Oil and egg tempera.

Size:
13 1/4" x 17"

Grateful appreciation is extended to Matt Bennett and the Marketing Communications Department at the U.S. Human Health Headquarters of Merck & Co., Inc. for their assistance and permission to reproduce the Paul Peck art·for the cover of this book.

No part of this book may be reproduced in any form or by any means, electronic or mechanical including photocopying, stored in an information retrieval system without the prior written permission of the Association of Medical Illustrators.

ISBN 1-883486-01-7, $50.00 USA

Editor:
William B. Westwood
Director of Marketing:
Linda Johnson

Source Book Editorial Board:
Christine D. Young, Chairperson
Don Biggerstaff
Nancy Chorpenning
Samuel Collins
Carrie Dilorenzo
Enid Hatton

Seventh Edition Design:
deCesare Design Associates
Darien, CT

Note:
All addresses and telephone numbers contained in this publication were correct at the time of printing, but people sometimes move. All artists can easily be located by call the Association of Medical Illustrators Headquarters at (800) 454-7900.

Copyright 1994 by the Association of Medical Illustrators. All rights reserved. Typeset and printed by Serbin Communications, Inc., Santa Barbara, CA.

For more information on the profession of Medical Illustration or any member please contact:

Association of Medical Illustrators
Association Headquarters
1819 Peachtree Street
Suite 712
Atlanta, GA 30309

(800) 454-7900
(404) 350-7900
Fax: (404) 351-3348

table of contents

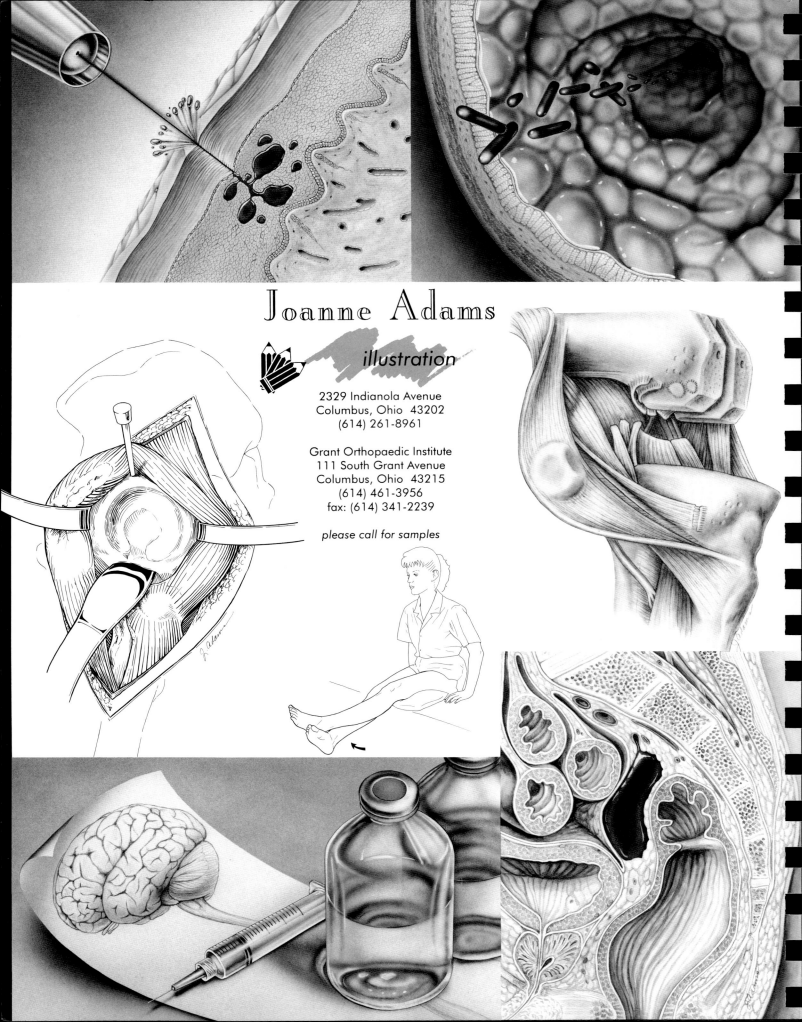

Joanne Adams

illustration

2329 Indianola Avenue
Columbus, Ohio 43202
(614) 261-8961

Grant Orthopaedic Institute
111 South Grant Avenue
Columbus, Ohio 43215
(614) 461-3956
fax: (614) 341-2239

please call for samples

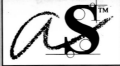

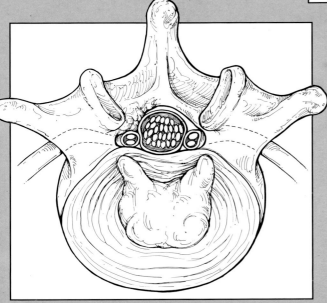

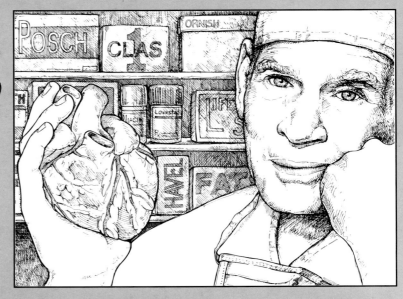

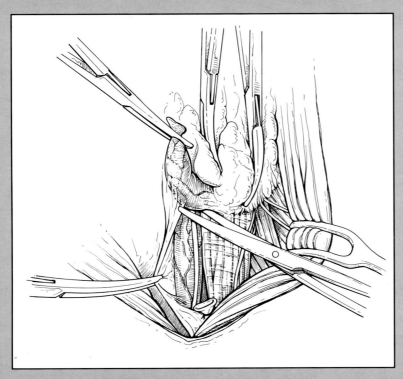

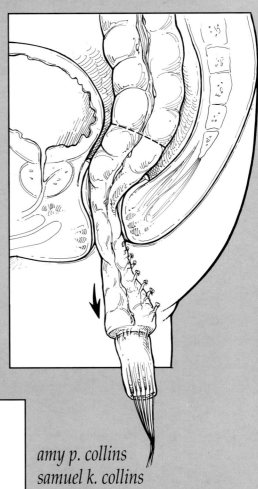

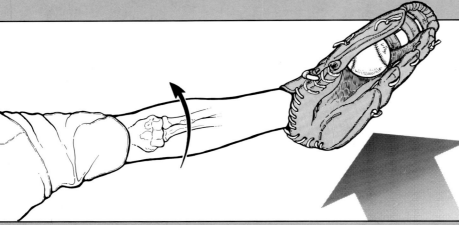

amy p. collins
samuel k. collins

art and science,®inc.
medical and graphic illustration

2815-A 18th Street South
Birmingham, AL 35209
(205) 871-4445
(205) 871-4465 fax

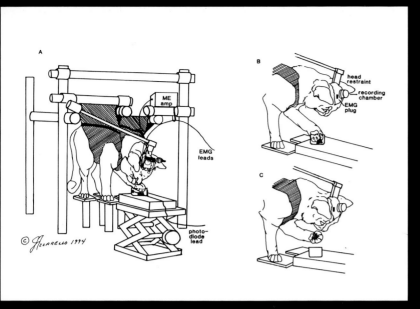

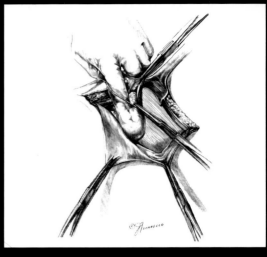

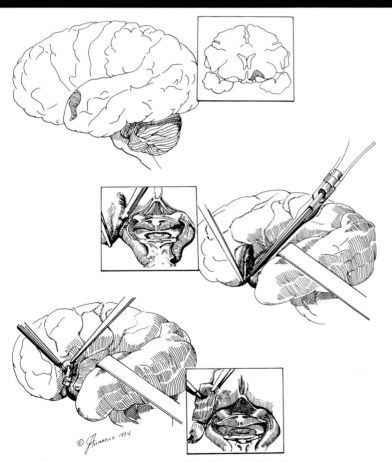

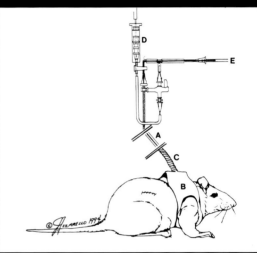

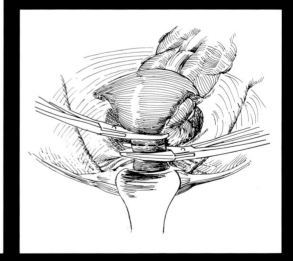

JAYNE AZZARELLO
every last detail
5455 N. Sheridan #2907
Chicago, IL 60640
(312) 878-4650

AREAS OF SPECIALIZATION: Zoological, Surgical, Anatomical Illustration in line and tone.

CLIENTS: Northwestern University Medical School, University of Chicago Medical School, Chicago Zoological Society, Montana State Department of Fish and Game, Raven Press.

PROFESSIONAL BACKGROUND: B.A. in Zoology with an emphasis in comparative reproductive physiology, endocrinology and anatomy, University of Montana. Artistic training at American Academy of Art, Chicago, and University of Illinois, Chicago.

PROFESSIONAL MEMBERSHIPS: Guild of Natural Science Illustrators.

AWARDS/HONORS: AMI/Vesalius Trust Research Grant For Graduate Research

The artist has 20 years combined experience in basic medical, biological, and zoological research with emphases on human and comparative neurobiology, reproductive biology and endocrinology.

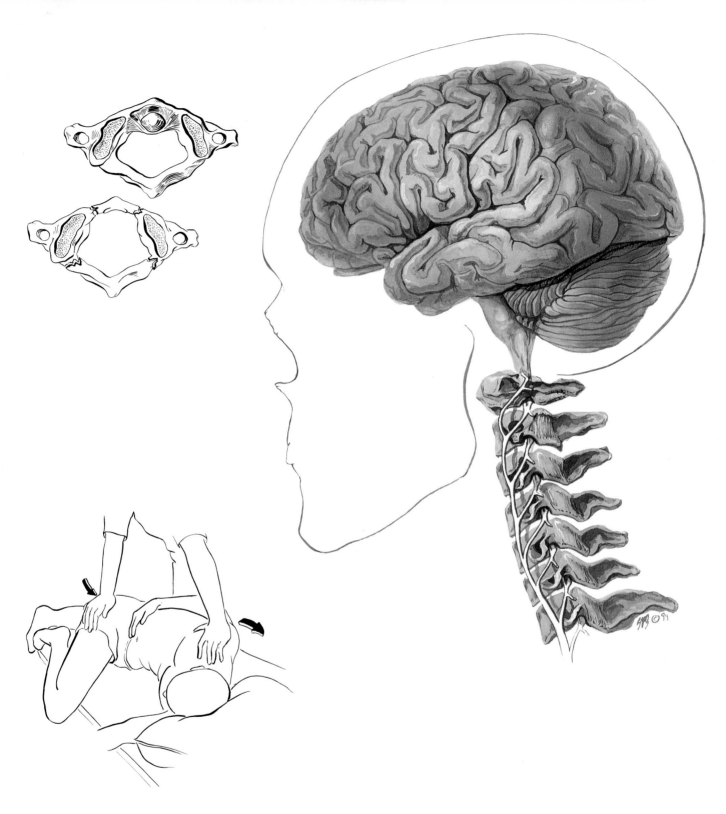

SYLVIA A. BLANKENSHIP, M.S.
HC67 Box 143
Floyd, VA 24091
Phone/FAX (703) 763-3377

AREAS OF SPECIALIZATION: Neuro-anatomy, Medical Testimony. Also veterinary and biomedical illustration for textbook and journal.

PROFESSIONAL BACKGROUND: M.S., Medical College of Georgia. B.F.A., The Rhode Island School of Design.

PROFESSIONAL MEMBERSHIPS: Association of Medical Illustrators, Guild of Natural Science Illustrators.

Virginia Hoyt Cantarella

Tel: 518-966-4419
Fax: 518-966-8375

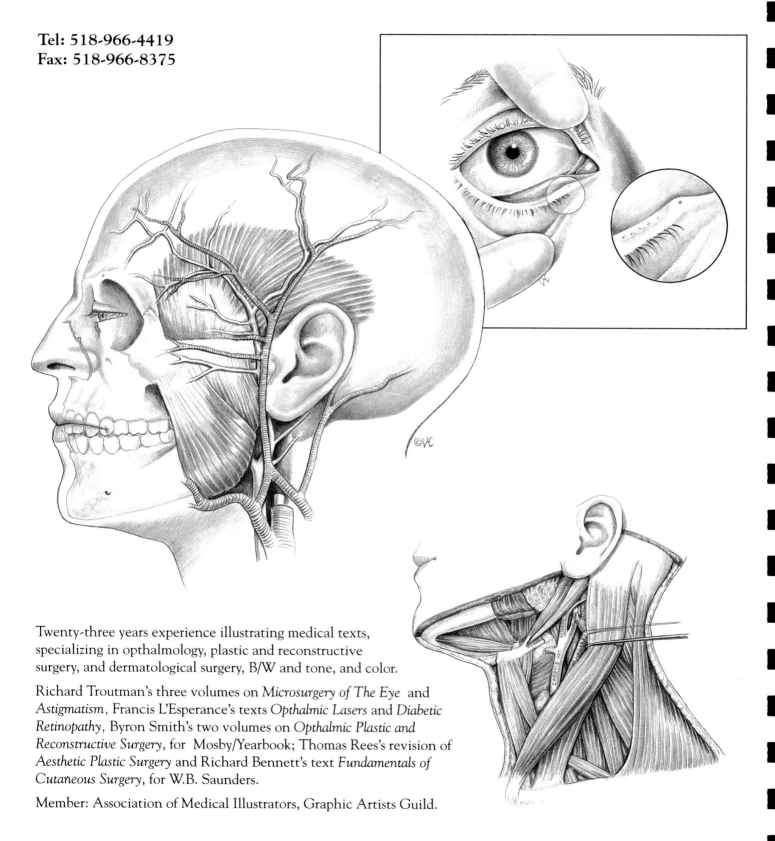

Twenty-three years experience illustrating medical texts, specializing in opthalmology, plastic and reconstructive surgery, and dermatological surgery, B/W and tone, and color.

Richard Troutman's three volumes on *Microsurgery of The Eye* and *Astigmatism*, Francis L'Esperance's texts *Opthalmic Lasers* and *Diabetic Retinopathy*, Byron Smith's two volumes on *Opthalmic Plastic and Reconstructive Surgery*, for Mosby/Yearbook; Thomas Rees's revision of *Aesthetic Plastic Surgery* and Richard Bennett's text *Fundamentals of Cutaneous Surgery*, for W.B. Saunders.

Member: Association of Medical Illustrators, Graphic Artists Guild.

P.O. Box 54, South Westerlo, New York 12163-0054

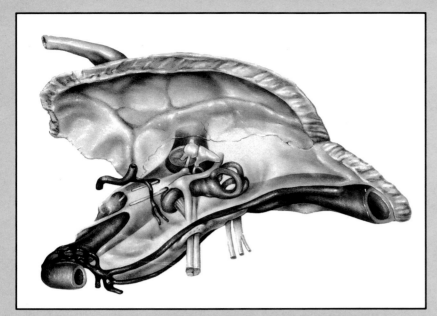

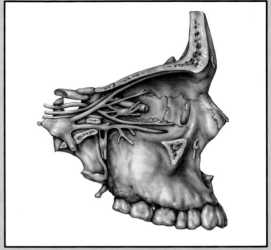

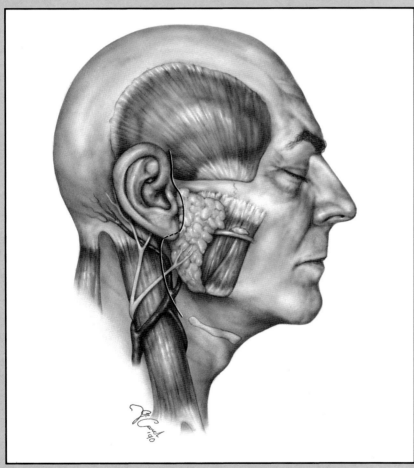

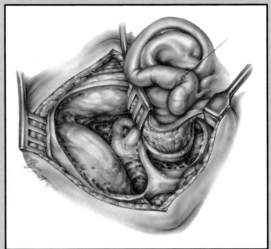

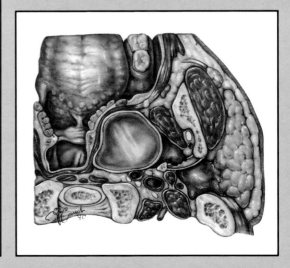

GEORGE CARD

Medical Art of Nashville
P.O. Box 808
Goodlettsville, TN 37072
Office (615) 329-7808 ext. 306
Home (615) 859-2804
FAX (615) 329-7935

AREAS OF SPECIALIZATION: Surgical, anatomical and conceptual illustrations in all types of media for use in medical publications and medical-legal courtroom presentations. Extensive experience in the field of otolaryngology—head and neck surgery.

CLIENTS: W.B. Saunders, Harcourt Brace Jovanovich, Churchill Livingstone, B.C. Decker, C.F. Mosby, John Wiley and Sons, Thieme-Stratton, Raven Press.

PROFESSIONAL BACKGROUND: M.S., Medical Illustration, Medical College of Georgia; Senior Staff Illustrator, University of Kentucky Medical Center; Section Chief of Medical Illustration and Photography, Meharry Medical College; Medical Illustrator, The EAR Foundation; extensive free-lance experience.

PROFESSIONAL MEMBERSHIPS: Association of Medical Illustrators.

AWARDS/HONORS: Sama Eaton Medical Art Salon, 2nd Place.

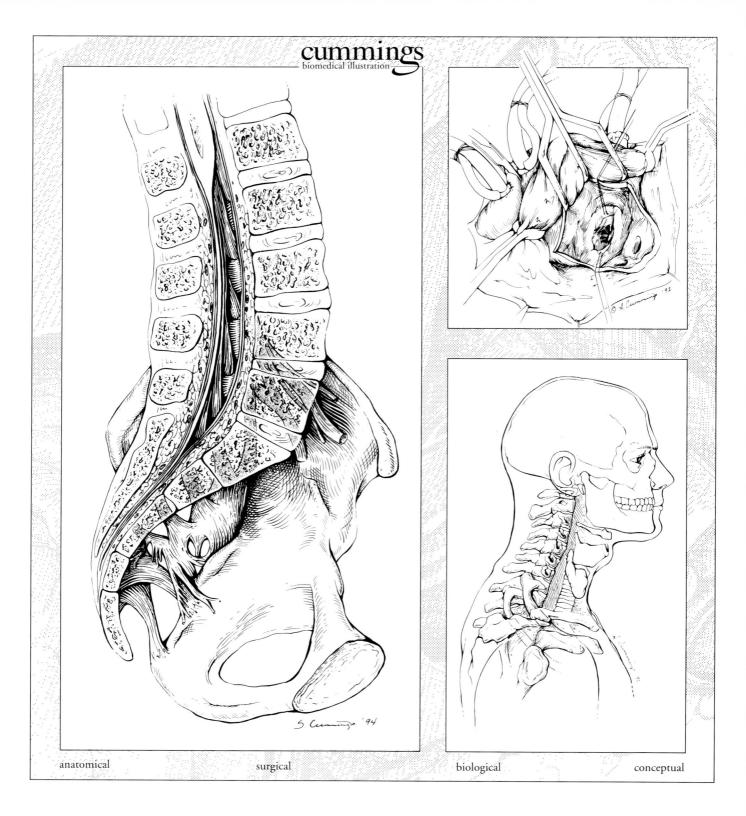

cummings
biomedical illustration

anatomical   surgical   biological   conceptual

SALLY CUMMINGS

Cummings Biomedical Illustration
18 West 078 Standish Lane
Villa Park, IL 60181
Phone/FAX (708) 627-7659
If contact is not made at the listed number,
please call the AMI headquarters at (404)
350-7900.

AREAS OF SPECIALIZATION: Anatomical,
surgical, biological, and conceptual illustration
for textbook and editorial use. Focused on,
but not limited to, spinal anatomy and neuro-
musculoskeletal system.

CLIENTS: Authors and publishers of medical
and scientific subject matter, including Mosby
Year Book, Inc., Aspen Publishing Co., Cliggott
Publishing Co., Anatomical Chart Co., Abbott
Laboratories, and Scientific American, as well as
numerous private health care physicians.

PROFESSIONAL BACKGROUND: B.A., Art
and Biology, State University of New York at
Potsdam, 1988. M.A.M.S., Biomedical Visualization, University of Illinois at Chicago, 1991.

Medical Illustrator (1.5 years), National College
of Chiropractic, Chicago, Illinois. Author and
Illustrator of *Understanding Trigger Points:
A Guide to Myofascial Pain and Discomfort.*
Freelance since 1991.

PROFESSIONAL MEMBERSHIPS: Association of Medical Illustrators, Midwest Medical
Illustrators.

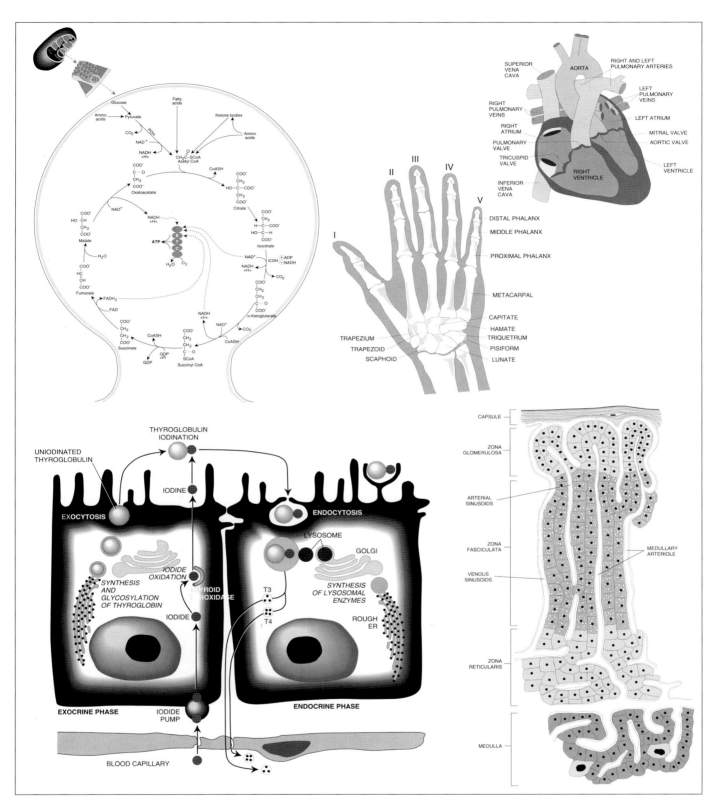

MOLLIE DUNKER

16525 Dubbs Road
Sparks, Maryland 21152
(410) 329-3871
FAX (410) 329-3183

AREAS OF SPECIALIZATION: Specializing in computer illustration for print and CD-ROM.

PROFESSIONAL BACKGROUND: B.A. in graphic design from the University of Illinois, Champaign-Urbana. Masters in Medical and Biological Illustration from Johns Hopkins University.

CLIENTS: Clients include WIlliams & Wilkins, Appleton-Lange, Lippincott, Johns Hopkins and Harvard Medical School staff physicians.

PROFESSIONAL MEMBERSHIPS: Member of the Association of Medical Illustrators, Audio-visual Management Association and International Television Association.

AWARDS/HONORS: Awards include an honorable mention for *Medical Genetics* at the 1992 American Medical Writers Association; first place, 1993 Maryland ITVA, training category for *Rosie's Rules for Handling White-Out;* honorable mention, 1993 Maryland ITVA, internal communications, for *We're Glad You Asked.*

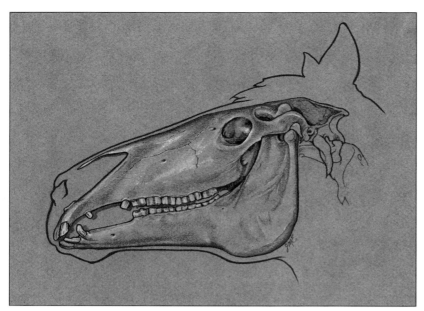

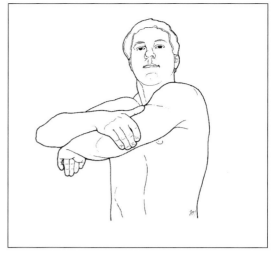

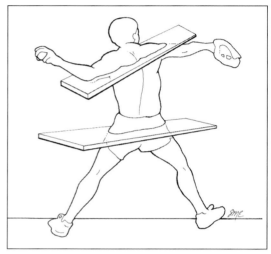

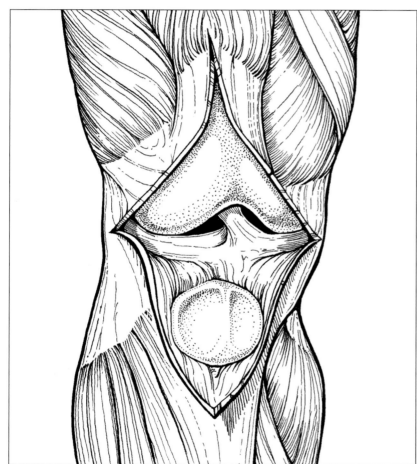

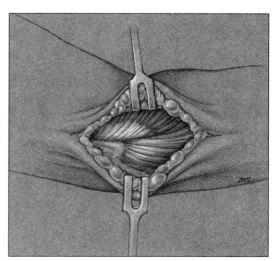

SUZANNE E.M. EDMONDS

2882 Shrider Road
Colorado Springs, CO 80920
(719) 528-8167

AREAS OF SPECIALIZATION: Anatomic, surgical, conceptual and diagrammatic visualizations of science and medicine. Particular specialization in orthopedic, sports medicine and biomechanic illustration.

CLIENTS: Mosby Yearbook; Williams and Wilkins; Howmedica; Intermedics Orthopedics; W.H. Freeman (*Scientific American*); *Western Horseman*; Aspen Publications; Kerlan-Jobe Orthopedic Clinic; The University of Southern California Center for Arthritis and Joint Implant Surgery; private physicians, surgeons and physical therapists.

PROFESSIONAL BACKGROUND: M.A. in Medcial and Biological Illustration, Johns Hopkins University School of Medicine; six years as Medical Illustrator at Centinela Hospital Medical Center, Inglewood, CA; Instructor of Anatomy and Pathology, The Stress Massage Institute (a school of massage therapy), Manitou Springs, CO.

PROFESSIONAL MEMBERSHIPS: The Association of Medical Illustrators.

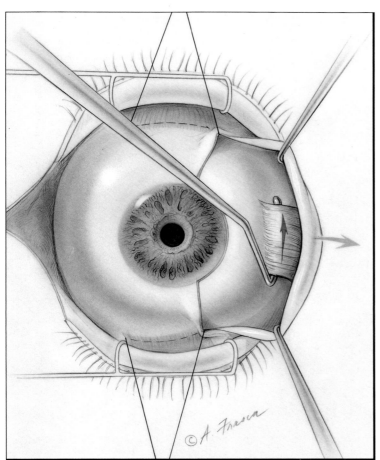

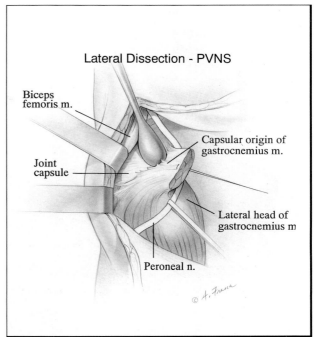

Lateral Dissection - PVNS

Biceps femoris m.

Capsular origin of gastrocnemius m.

Joint capsule

Lateral head of gastrocnemius m

Peroneal n.

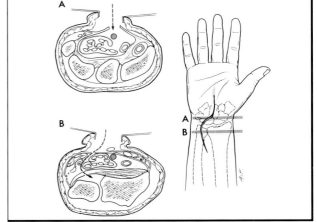

A

B

VERTEBROBASILAR CIRCULATION

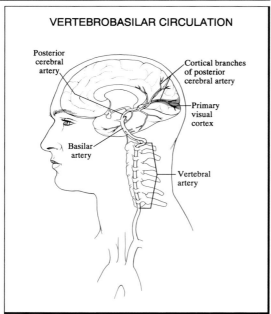

Posterior cerebral artery

Cortical branches of posterior cerebral artery

Primary visual cortex

Basilar artery

Vertebral artery

ARLEEN FRASCA

MEDICAL/ BIOMEDICAL ILLUSTRATION

(617) 662-4263

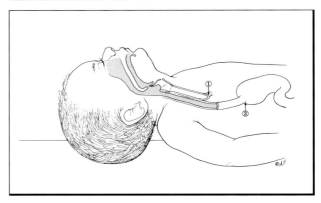

ARLEEN FRASCA
5 Garfield Road
Melrose, MA 02176
Phone/FAX (617) 662-4263

AREAS OF SPECIALIZATION: Continuous tone, line, color illustration for medical and lay audience. Illustration for surgical, textbook and trade publications. Conceptual illustrations for advertising and medical-legal exhibits.

CLIENTS: Publishers include W.B. Saunders, Williams and Wilkins, J.B. Lippincott, Springer-Verlag, Readers Digest Publications, Simon & Schuster. Corporate clients include Porex Surgi-cal, John Boswell Associates, William Douglas McAdams, Boston area law firms.

PROFESSIONAL BACKGROUND: BFA, Rhode Island School of Design, Illustration. MFA, University of Michigan, Medical and Biological Illustration.

PROFESSIONAL MEMBERSHIPS: Association of Medical Illustrators.

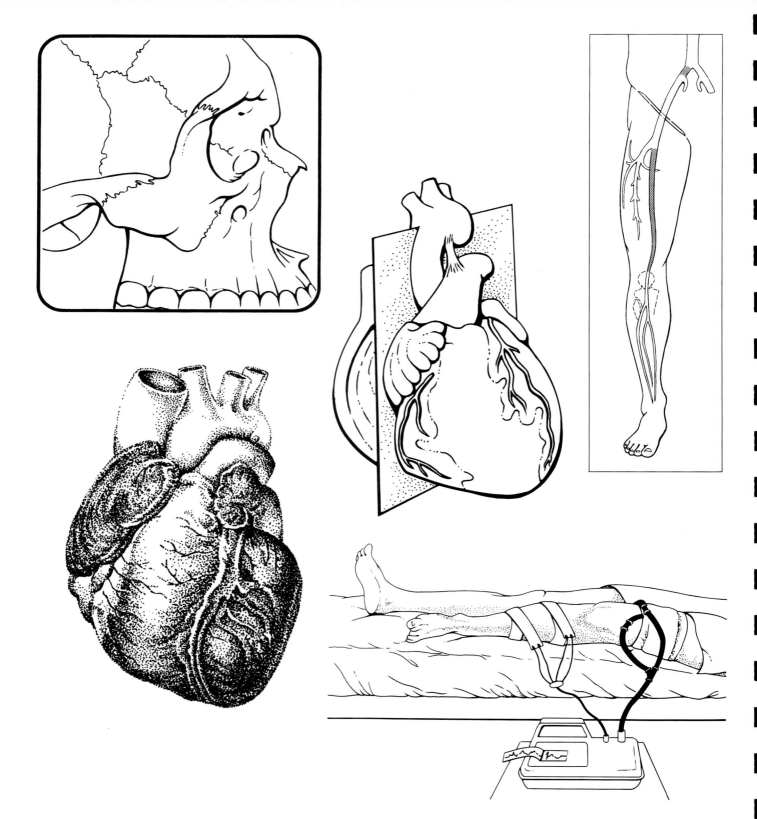

PATRICIA GAST
Medical Illustrator
163 Johnson Road
Scarsdale, NY 10583
(914) 723-0489

AREAS OF SPECIALIZATION: Medical illustration in pen-and-ink and computer graphic format for educational markets.

CLIENTS: Medical textbook and atlas publishers including Raven Press, Gower Medical Publishing, and Mosby-Yearbook, Inc.

PROFESSIONAL BACKGROUND: Freelance Illustrator; Staff Illustrator, Gower Medical Publishing.

PROFESSIONAL MEMBERSHIPS: Association of Medical Illustrators.

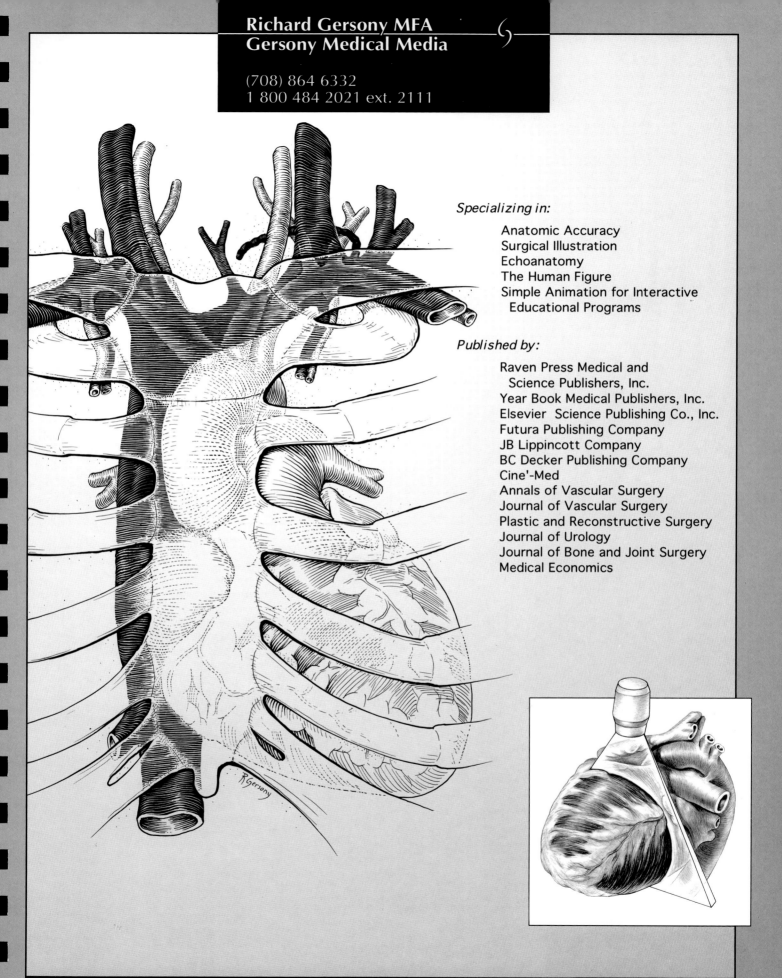

Richard Gersony MFA
Gersony Medical Media

(708) 864 6332
1 800 484 2021 ext. 2111

Specializing in:

Anatomic Accuracy
Surgical Illustration
Echoanatomy
The Human Figure
Simple Animation for Interactive
  Educational Programs

Published by:

Raven Press Medical and
  Science Publishers, Inc.
Year Book Medical Publishers, Inc.
Elsevier Science Publishing Co., Inc.
Futura Publishing Company
JB Lippincott Company
BC Decker Publishing Company
Cine'-Med
Annals of Vascular Surgery
Journal of Vascular Surgery
Plastic and Reconstructive Surgery
Journal of Urology
Journal of Bone and Joint Surgery
Medical Economics

Certified by the Association of Medical Illustrators and Winner of the Russell Drake Award of Exellence for Medical Line 1992

HAKOLA STUDIO

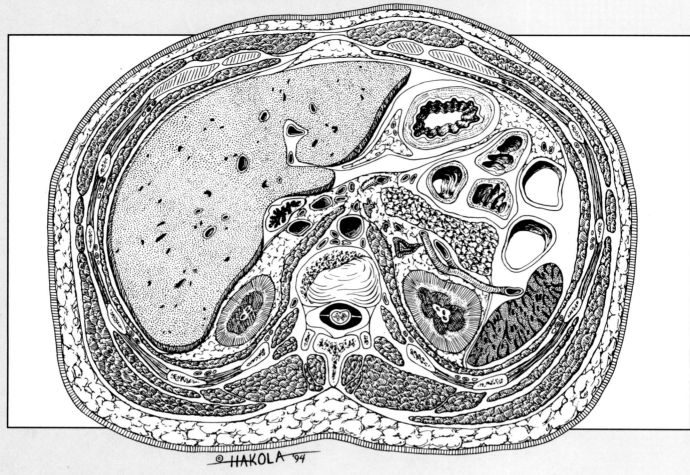

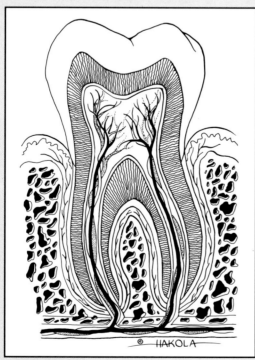

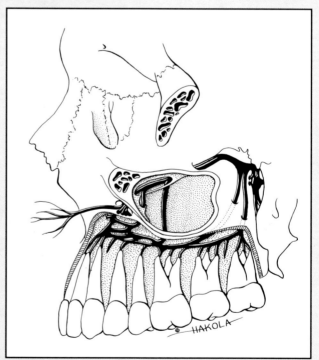

SUSAN HAKOLA

Medical and Scientific Illustration

16990 Martin-Welch Road
Marysville, Ohio 43040
(513) 642-2837

Illustration key, clockwise from top:

1. Abdominal cross-section at the level of T-12
2. Anatomy of superior dental nerve plexus
3. Schematic cross-section of a lower molar

Curriculum vitae and portfolio samples available on request.

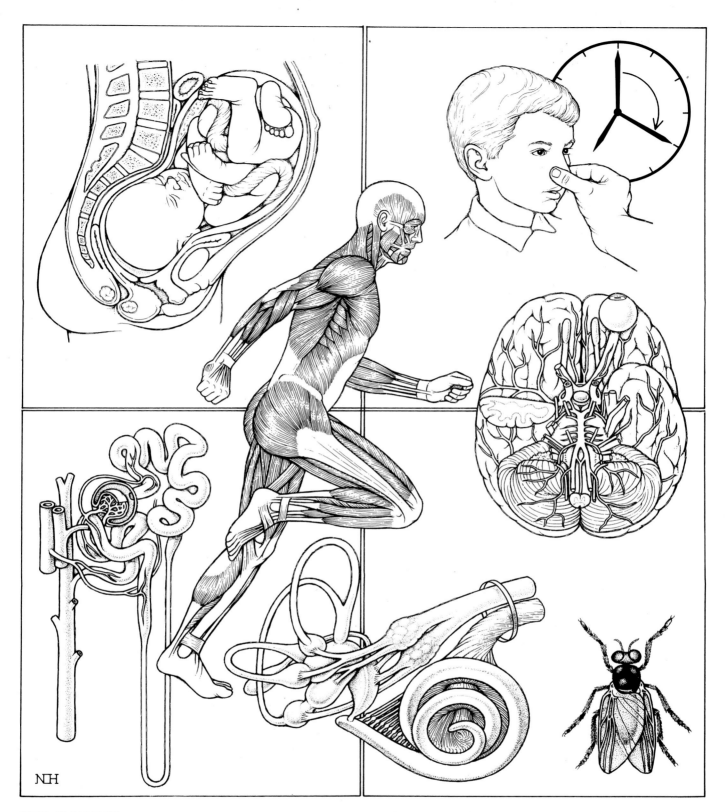

NEIL O. HARDY

Two Woods Grove Road
Westport, CT 06880
Phone/FAX (203) 226-4446

AREAS OF SPECIALIZATION: Surgical, anatomical, physiological and molecular illustrations in line, tone and color for medicine and biology.

CLIENTS: Scientific American, New York Times, Esquire Magazine, Readers Digest, American Heritage Dictionary, American Journal of Nursing, Modern Medicine Magazine, Advances in Oncology, H.I.V. Advances in Research and Therapy, McGraw-Hill, Time Inc.

PROFESSIONAL BACKGROUND: Assistant Professor, Art as Applied to Medicine, The Johns Hopkins University School of Medicine; B.F.A., The Maryland College of Art; three-year certificate in medical illustration from The Johns Hopkins University School of Medicine.

PROFESSIONAL MEMBERSHIPS: The Association of Medical Illustrators, The New York Society of Illustrators, The Graphic Artists Guild, The Guild of Natural Science Illustrators.

AWARDS/HONORS: The Ranice W. Crosby Distinguished Achievement Award from The Johns Hopkins University School of Medicine, 1991; Best Illustrated Medical Book Award, A.M.I. 1976; 2nd place Medical Line Illustration, A.M.I. 1976; Honorable Mention Medical Line Illustration, Bio 84 meeting; first place, Medical and Scientific Illustration, Mid-Atlantic Bio Communications, 1985.

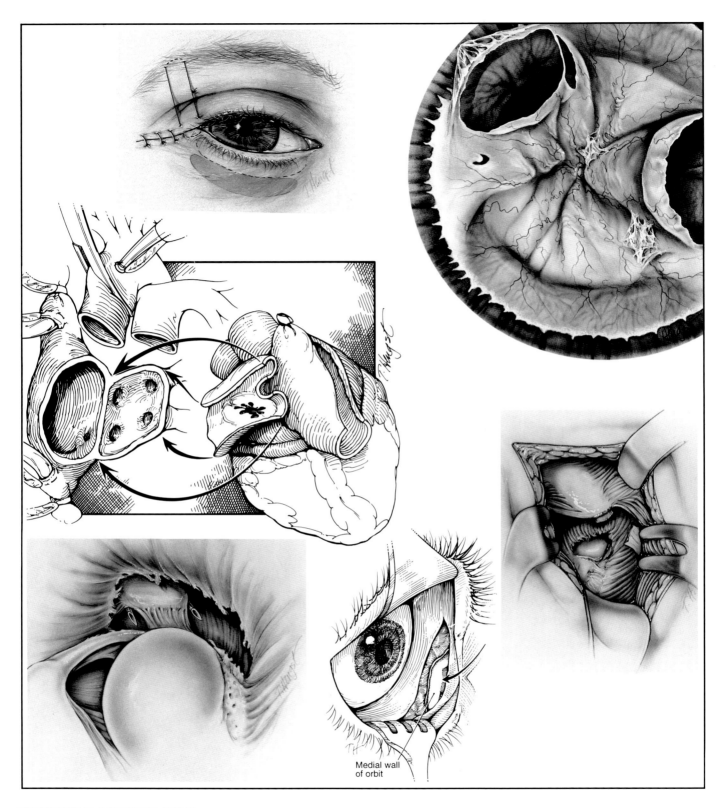

Medial wall
of orbit

TIMOTHY C. HENGST, FAMI

T.C. Hengst & Associates
1631 Calle de Oro
Thousand Oaks, CA 91360
(805) 523-0268
FAX (805) 523-1139

AREAS OF SPECIALIZATION: Illustrated over fifteen volumes in ophthalmology. Significant experience in cardiovascular, orthopedic and plastic surgery. Instructional, anatomical, surgical and technical illustration for medical publishing.

CLIENTS: Lea & Febiger, Mosby/Yearbook, J.B. Lippincott Co., Walt Disney Imagineering, Doheny Eye Institute–USC, Jules Stein Eye Institute–UCLA, Ace Medical Company, Baxter Healthcare Corp., private physicians and surgeons.

PROFESSIONAL BACKGROUND: M.A. in Medical & Biological Illustration, Johns Hopkins University School of Medicine; three years at Texas Heart Institute; nine years on faculty at Johns Hopkins; freelance since 1986.

PROFESSIONAL MEMBERSHIPS: Association of Medical Illustrators, Society of Illustrators of Los Angeles.

AWARDS/HONORS: AMI Illustrated Medical Book Awards in 1980, 1990, and 1993; AMI Russel Drake Award 1993 and numerous other AMI salon awards.

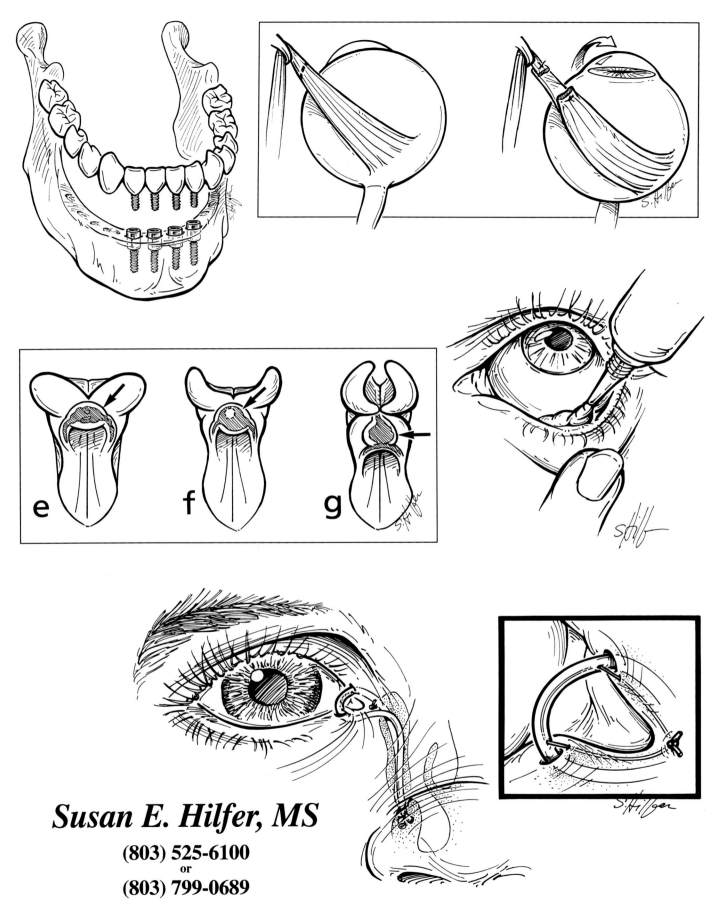

Susan E. Hilfer, MS

(803) 525-6100
or
(803) 799-0689

Medical Illustration
medical / legal ◆ surgical ◆ anatomical ◆ conceptual

Nematode and Body Parts

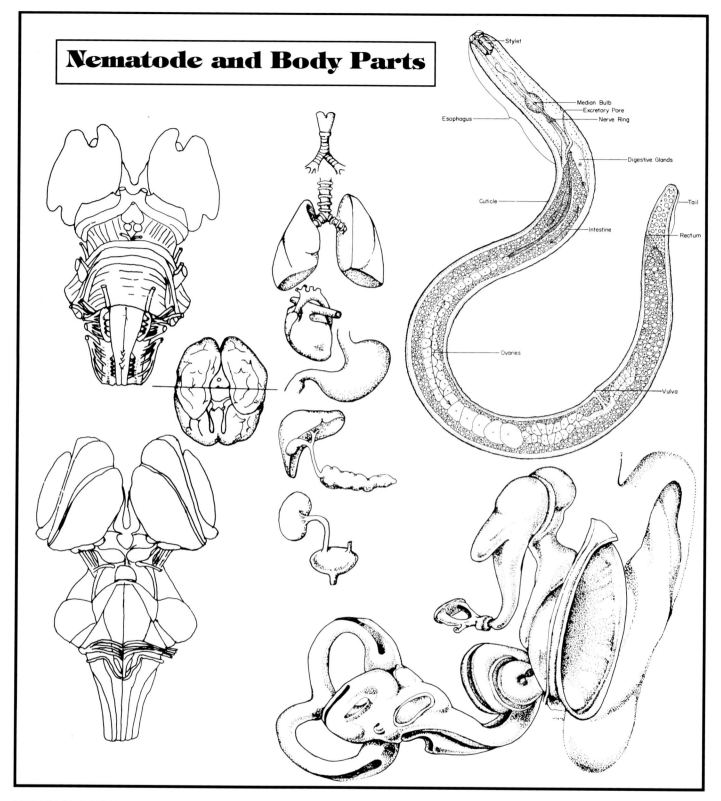

Stylet
Median Bulb
Excretory Pore
Nerve Ring
Esophagus
Digestive Glands
Cuticle
Tail
Intestine
Rectum
Ovaries
Vulva

HELEN K. HUSEMAN
1739 S.W. Rocky Pt. Rd.
Gainesville, FL 32608
(904) 372-6176
FAX (904) 392-8583

AREAS OF SPECIALIZATION: Conceptual and general medical illustration in line, color or tone for print or projected media; also, exhibit design and desktop publishing.

CLIENTS: Maupin House Publishers, Shands Teaching Hospital, College of Veterinary Medicine (University of Florida), Dept. of Microbiological & Cell Science, Asso. in Physical Therapy.

PROFESSIONAL BACKGROUND: B.A. in Commercial Art from Memphis College of Art, Grant School of Design and independent studies in medical, biological and botanical illustration, 22 years as senior illustrator for the Institute of Food & Agricultural Sciences.

PROFESSIONAL MEMBERSHIPS: Association of Medical Illustrators, Guild of Natural Science Illustrators and Agricultural Communicators in Education.

WENDY BETH JACKELOW

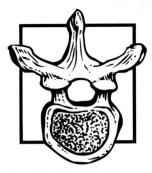

Medical & Scientific Illustration

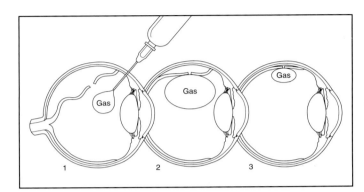

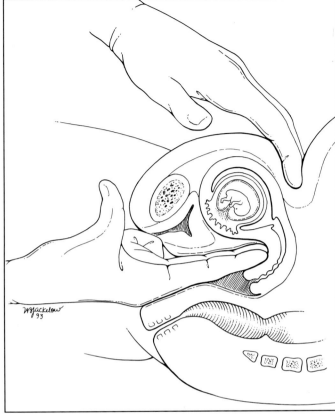

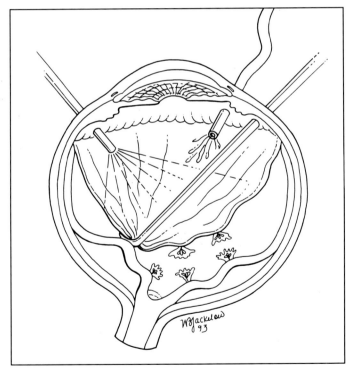

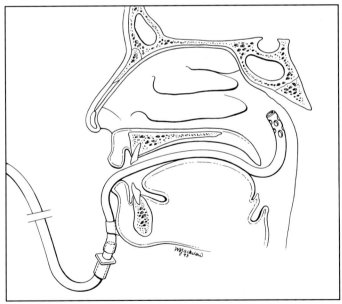

WENDY BETH JACKELOW
Medical & Scientific Illustration
266 Pelton Avenue
Staten Island, New York 10310
Phone/FAX (718) 273-0002

AREAS OF SPECIALIZATION: Medical and scientific illustration and design for textbooks and publications. Emphasis is on production of quality illustrations within budget and on time for assignments large or small. Also specializing in computer illustration, charts and graphs.

PROFESSIONAL BACKGROUND: M.F.A. in Medical Illustration, Rochester Institute of Technology. B.A. in Biology, University of Rochester.

PROFESSIONAL MEMBERSHIPS: Association of Medical Illustrators, Guild of Natural Science Illustrators.

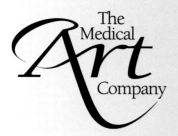

The Medical **Art** Company

Contact Marcia Hartsock, CMI
2142 Alpine Place
Cincinnati, Ohio 45206-2603
TEL 513 221-3868
FAX 513 221-3859

Quality Standards
• Clear, concise images
• Scientific accuracy
• Elegant style
• On-time delivery

National Clients
• Churchill Livingstone, Inc.
• Krames Communications
• Marion Merrell Dow
• Medical Economics Publishers
• Ortho Pharmaceuticals
• Procter & Gamble
• W.C. Brown Publishers
• Williams & Wilkins

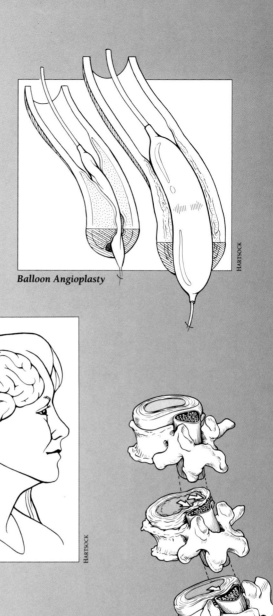

Balloon Angioplasty

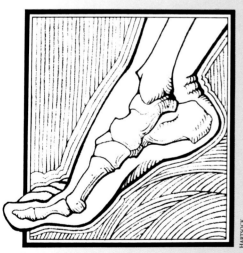

Bones of the Foot

Origin of Partial Seizures

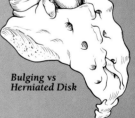

**Bulging vs
Herniated Disk**

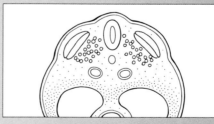

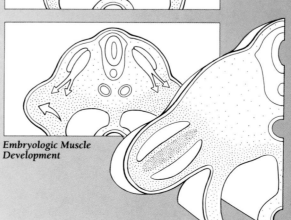

**Embryologic Muscle
Development**

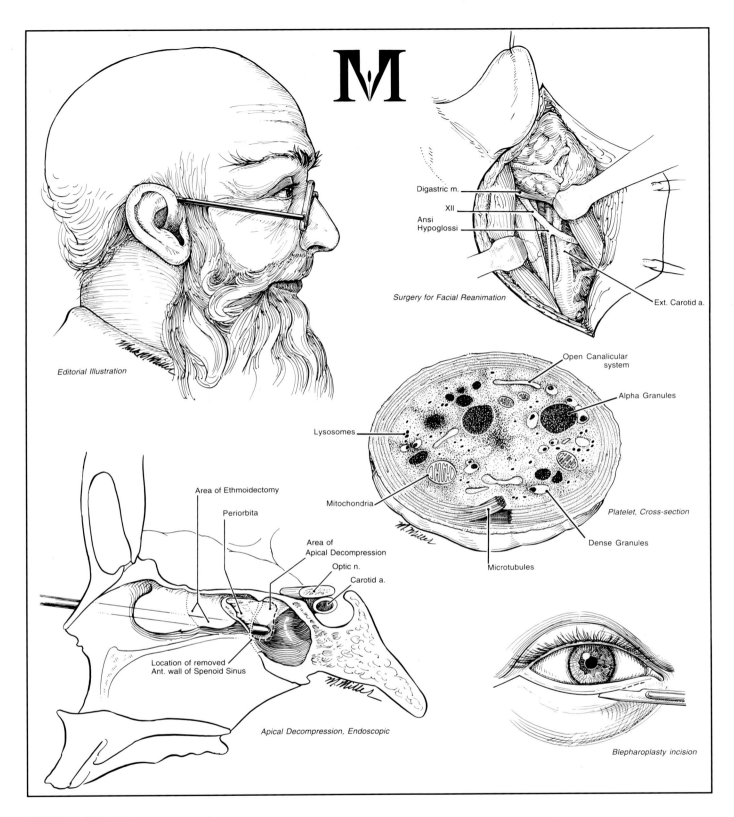

Editorial Illustration

Digastric m.

XII

Ansi Hypoglossi

Surgery for Facial Reanimation

Ext. Carotid a.

Open Canalicular system

Alpha Granules

Lysosomes

Mitochondria

Platelet, Cross-section

Dense Granules

Microtubules

Area of Ethmoidectomy

Periorbita

Area of Apical Decompression

Optic n.

Carotid a.

Location of removed Ant. wall of Spenoid Sinus

Apical Decompression, Endoscopic

Blepharoplasty incision

MARK M. MILLER

P.O. Box 422
Liberty, Missouri 64068
Phone/FAX (816) 792-2671

AREAS OF SPECIALIZATION: Surgical, anatomic and conceptual illustration in traditional pen & ink or electronic media. Special interest and expertise in the anatomy and surgery of the head and neck. Color illustration and medical models.

CLIENTS: Mosby Year Book, Blackwell Scientific Publishing, Thieme Medical Publishers, Inc., Chapman & Hall, J.B. Lippincott Co., Simulaids, Inc., Archives of Otolaryngology/Head and Neck Surgery, Laryngoscope and numerous medical and legal professionals.

PROFESSIONAL BACKGROUND: M.A. in Medical and Biological Illustration from the Johns Hopkins University School of Medicine, Department of Art as Applied to Medicine. Five years experience as an Instructor and Illustrator

in Art as Applied to Medicine. Currently a part-time Instructor in Art as Applied to Medicine.

PROFESSIONAL MEMBERSHIPS: Active Member of the A.M.I. (1987).

Shavell

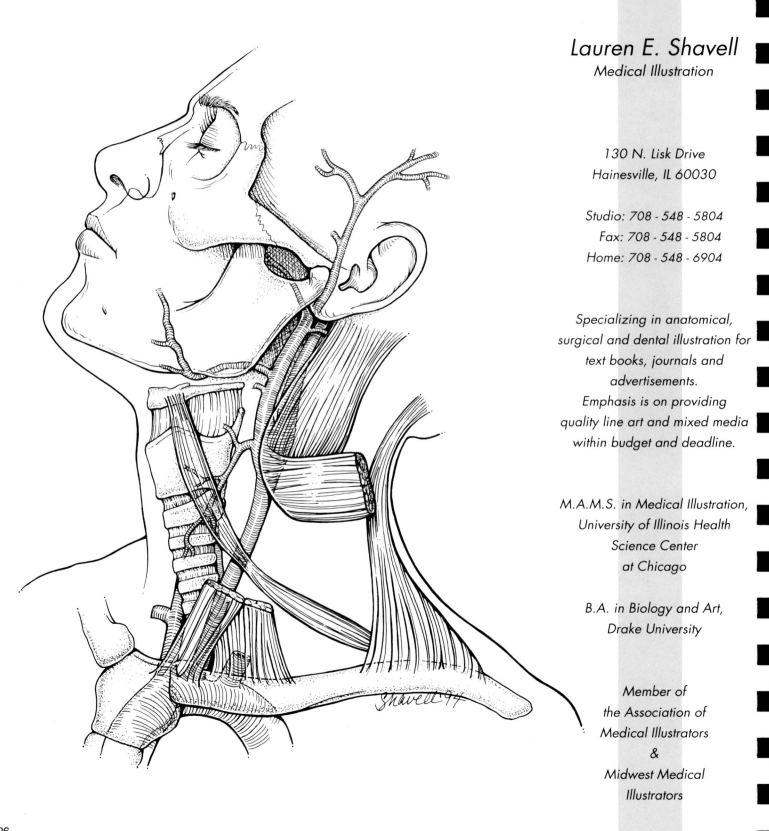

Lauren E. Shavell
Medical Illustration

130 N. Lisk Drive
Hainesville, IL 60030

Studio: 708 - 548 - 5804
Fax: 708 - 548 - 5804
Home: 708 - 548 - 6904

Specializing in anatomical,
surgical and dental illustration for
text books, journals and
advertisements.
Emphasis is on providing
quality line art and mixed media
within budget and deadline.

M.A.M.S. in Medical Illustration,
University of Illinois Health
Science Center
at Chicago

B.A. in Biology and Art,
Drake University

Member of
the Association of
Medical Illustrators
&
Midwest Medical
Illustrators

PAT THOMAS

MEDICAL ILLUSTRATION

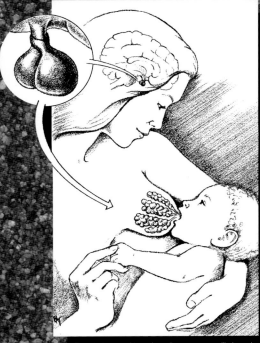

The pituitary and lactation – line art on coquille board

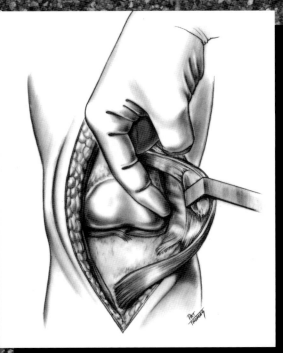

Lateral release of knee ligaments

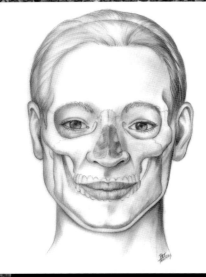

Relationships of bony support

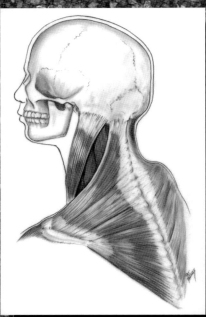

The trapezius muscle

Board certified; Graduate of University of Illinois Medical Illustration program, with honors

Over 20 years of time & budget efficient illustration in one, two and four color

Textbook titles in orthopedics, nursing, physical assessment, neuroanatomy, anatomy and other disciplines

Pat Thomas, CMI
Pat Thomas Medical Illustration
711 Carpenter
Oak Park, IL 60604-1106
708-383-8505
fax 708-383-8551

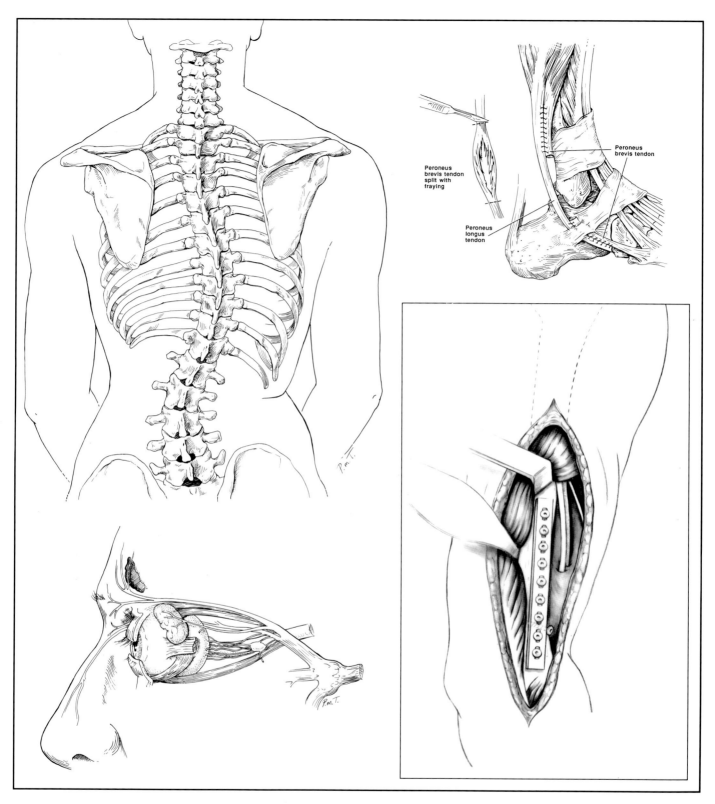

Peroneus brevis tendon split with fraying

Peroneus longus tendon

Peroneus brevis tendon

PAULINE M. THOMAS
965 Lexington Avenue
New York, NY 10021
(212) 744-3198
FAX Available

AREAS OF SPECIALIZATION: Surgical and anatomical illustration in line, tone, and color, for medical textbooks, magazines, journals and advertising. Special interest in orthopaedic surgery and veterinary medicine.

CLIENTS: The New York Hospital–Cornell Medical Center, The Hospital for Special Surgery, The Animal Medical Center, *Hospital Practice* Magazine, *Scientific American*, Williams & Wilkins, J.B. Lipincott Co., McGraw Hill and numerous private physicians.

PROFESSIONAL MEMBERSHIPS: Association of Medical Illustrators, Graphic Artists Guild, Institute of Medical Illustrators.

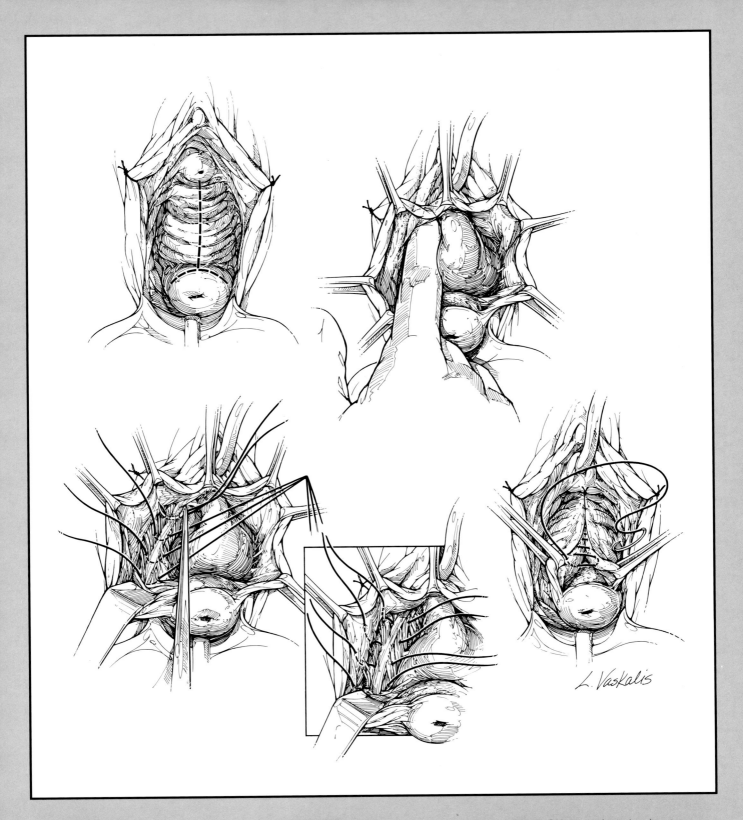

L. Vaskalis

LORI VASKALIS
134 S.E. 76th Avenue
Portland, OR 97215-1464
(503) 252-5552
FAX (503) 252-0874

ILLUSTRATION: B&W line and mixed media/ color illustration for surgical texts, juvenile publications, and presentation graphics.

ANIMATION: Quantel Paintbox/Harriet animation created for clients in the pharmaceutical, educational, and equipment manufacturing industries. Video Demo Reel available upon request.

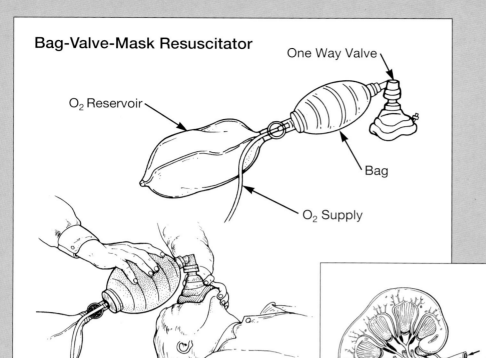

Bag-Valve-Mask Resuscitator

One Way Valve

O₂ Reservoir

Bag

O₂ Supply

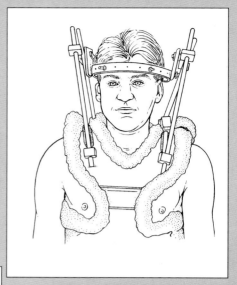

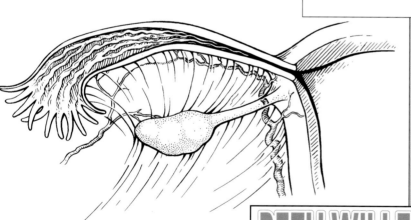

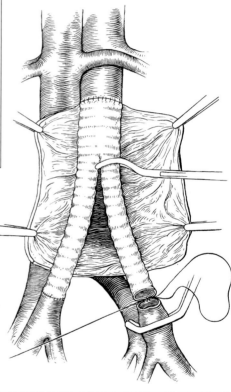

AREAS OF SPECIALIZATION: B&W, continuous tone and color work for anatomical, biological, clinical, product and technical illustration. Line illustration styles range from simple, linear depictions to complex, modeled images for textbooks, journals, manuals, magazines, projection media, posters, advertising and medical legal use.

CLIENTS: Abbott Labs, Berlex, Bristol Myers Squibb, Carter Wallace, Ethicon, Johnson & Johnson, Pfizer, Sandoz, Schering-Plough, Churchill Livingstone, F.A. Davis, Harper Collins, Medical Economics Company, numerous ad agencies, physicians and attorneys.

**BETH WILLERT
M.S.
MEDICAL
ILLUSTRATOR**

4 Woodland Drive, Roselle, NJ 07203

(908) 298-1237 • Fax (908) 298-9148

PROFESSIONAL BACKGROUND: B.A., Art, and B.S., Biology, Michigan State University. M.S., Medical and Biological Illustration, University of Michigan. Two-year staff position, Children's Hospital National Medical Center in Washington, D.C. Freelance since 1982. Board Certified.

PROFESSIONAL MEMBERSHIPS: Association of Medical Illustrators, Graphic Artists Guild 1983-1993, Guild of Natural Science Illustrators, Society of Illustrators-New York.

© Beth Willert, 1994

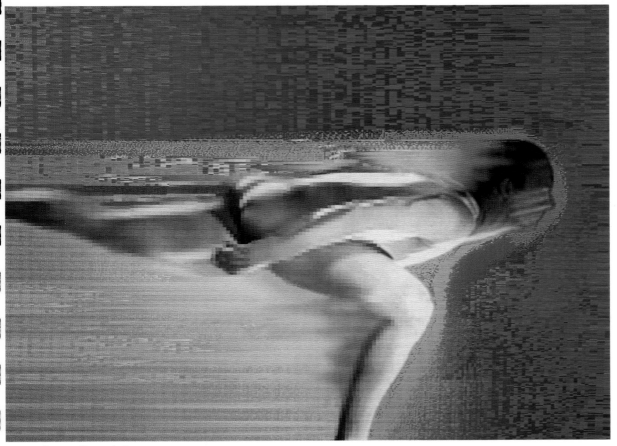

Schering/Ferguson Communications

AHI REPRESENTS

SHARMEN
LIAO
i n c.

COMPUTER
ILLUSTRATION
818 · 458 · 7699

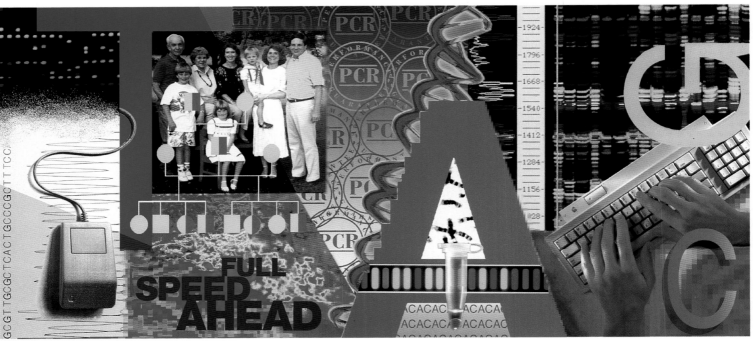

Applied Biosystems

AHI

108 East 35 St.
New York 10016
(212) 889-3337
Fax: (212) 889-3341

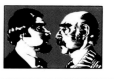

ART FOR THE HEALTHCARE INDUSTRY

A DIVISION OF
GERALD & CULLEN RAPP INC.

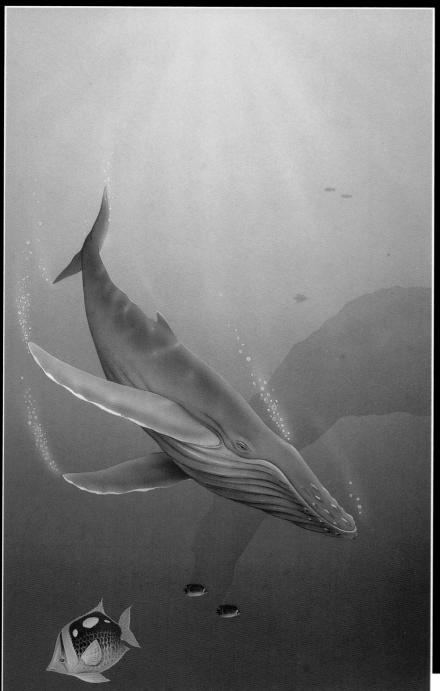

Absolute Science

Carlyn Iverson

(612) 645-7508
515 Glendale St.
St. Paul, MN
55104

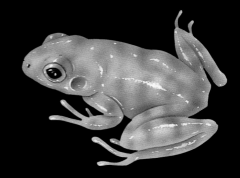

Full-color conceptual illustration created for science publications including: college and medical textbooks, science-related magazines, and advertising. Also encyclopedia and children's publications.

accuracy

aesthetics

drama

clarity

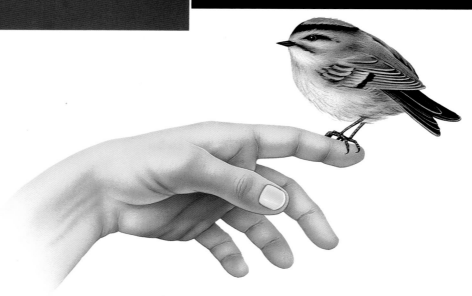

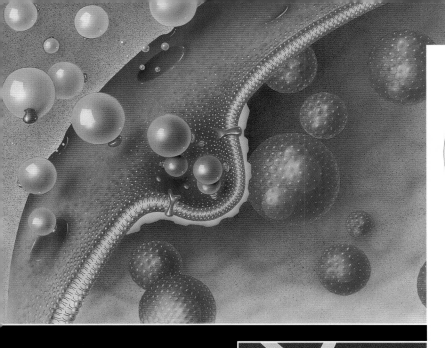

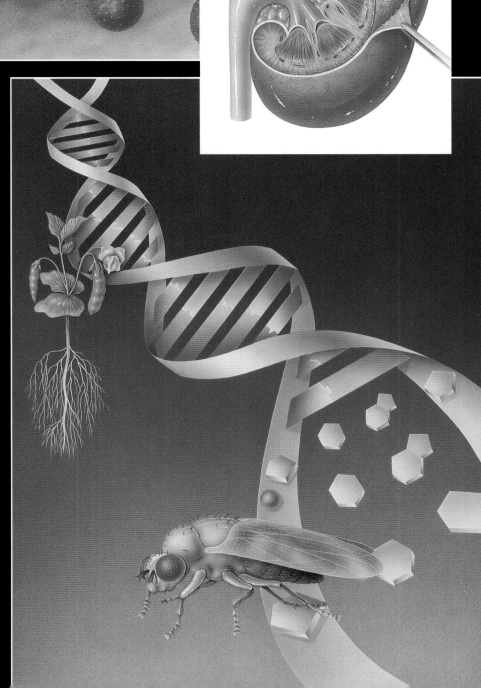

Subject sampling:

biology
anatomy
genetics
microbiology
oceanography
environmental science
molecular biology
psychology
physiology
zoology
geology
botany

Client sampling:

Brown Communications
Scientific American
John Wiley & Sons
West Publishing
W.H. Freeman
Saunders
Mosby
Wadsworth
McGraw-Hill
Times-Mirror
Raven Medical
Addison-Wesley

SLIDE & TEARSHEET SAMPLES
PROVIDED ON REQUEST

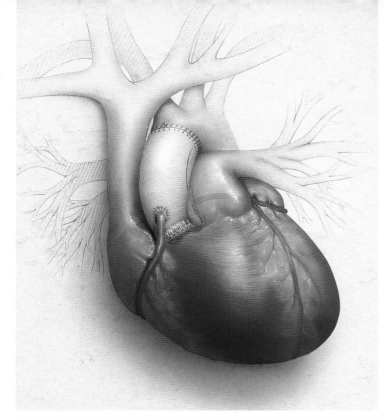
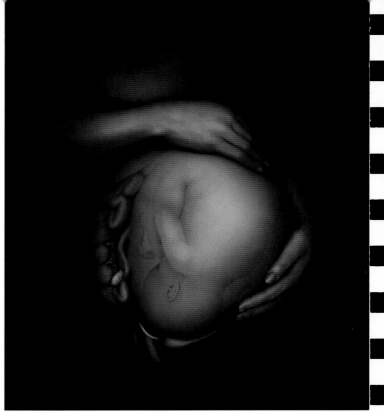
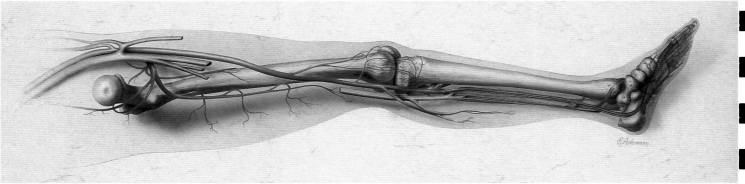
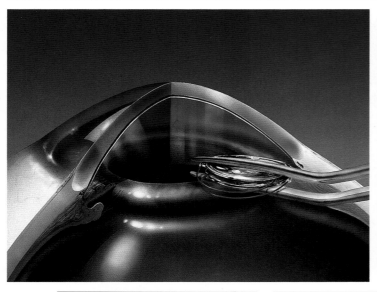
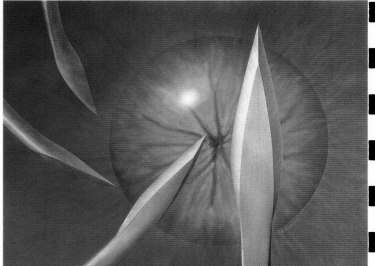

RODD AMBROSON, B.F.A., M.A.

141 N. State St., #215
Lake Oswego, OR 97034
TEL: **(503) 635-6238** FAX: (503) 635-7040

EXPERIENCE:
Freelance medical illustration 1987 to present. M.A., University of Texas Health Science Center, 1985. B.F.A., Oregon State University, 1980. Adjunct Professor of Art: Portland State University, 1987 - 1990; Marylhurst College, 1990 to present.

AREA OF SPECIALIZATION:
While providing creative solutions for advertising agencies, design firms and biomedical product companies, Rodd brings a quality to projects that elevates medical illustration to an art form.

AnatomyWorks Inc.

Stock Medical Illustrations

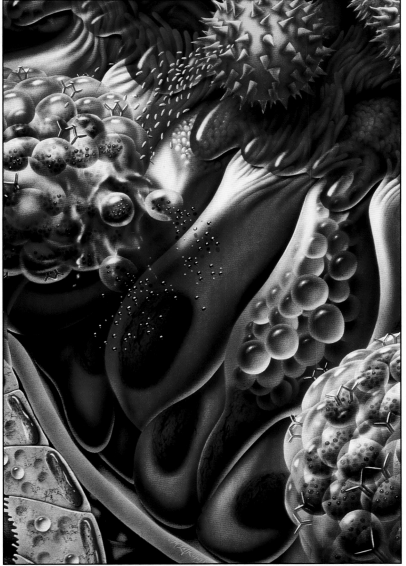

MARK LEFKOWITZ/
ALLERGIC RESPONSE

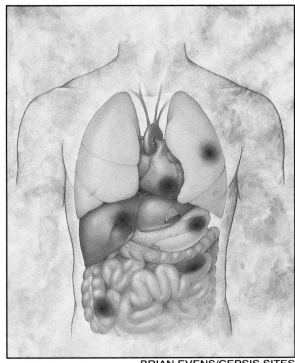

BRIAN EVENS/CEPSIS SITES

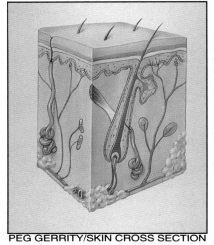

PEG GERRITY/SKIN CROSS SECTION

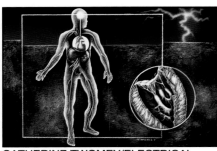

CATHERINE TWOMEY/ELECTRICAL
STIMULATION OF HEART

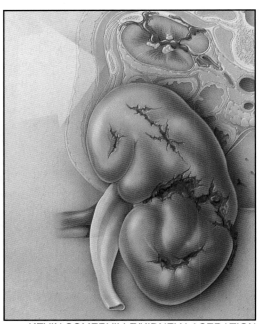

KEVIN SOMERVILLE/KIDNEY LACERATION

232 Madison Avenue New York, NY 10016
212/679-8480 ☎ 800/233-1975 ☎ Fax: 212/532-1934

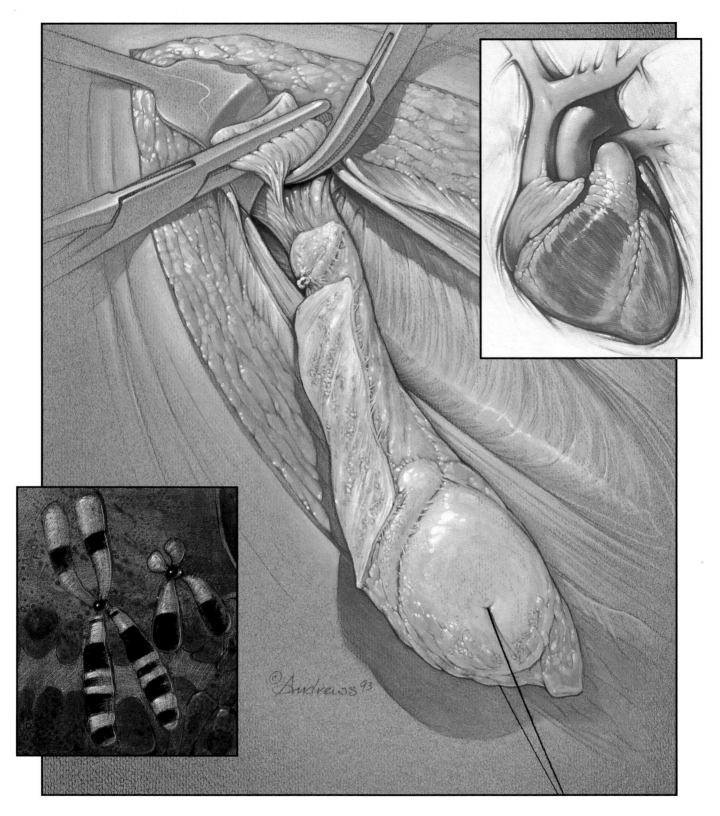

©Andrews 93

BILL ANDREWS, MA, CMI, FAMI

Bill Andrews & Associates, Inc.
Post Office Box 300885
Medical Center Station
Houston, TX 77230-0885
(713) 668-8897

AREAS OF SPECIALIZATION: Cancer, the Lymphatic System, the Cardiovascular System and Cardiothoracic Surgery, Diagnostic and Interventional Cardiology, Gynecology, Breast Surgery, Head and Neck Surgery, Urology and Prostate Surgery.

CLIENTS: Works are commissioned by a variety of clients across the country for advertising, editorial, clinical instruction, marketing, and patient education uses.

STOCK ART: Selected images are available through The Image Bank, Inc.

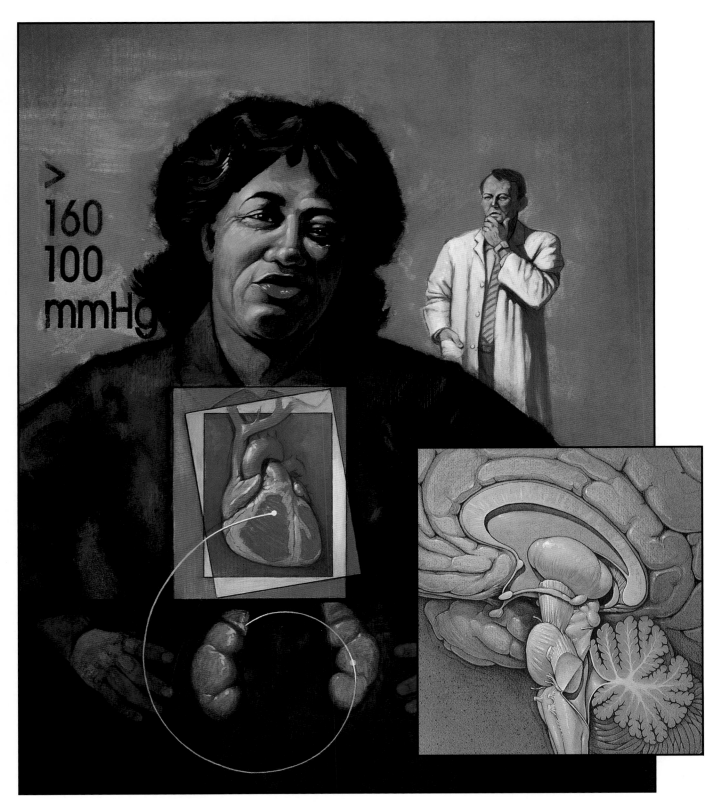

PROFESSIONAL BACKGROUND: Over 12 years professional experience using visual problem-solving skills and creativity to produce organic, soft-tech illustrations for advertising, editorial and marketing clients nationwide.

PROFESSIONAL MEMBERSHIPS: Association of Medical Illustrators and Graphic Artists Guild

SELECTED AWARDS: Ralph Sweet, Will Shepard and Russell Drake Awards from the Association of Medical Illustrators; Gold and Silver Medals from the Houston Society of Illustrators; Gold and Silver Medals from the Society of Illustrators of Los Angeles

BILL ANDREWS, MA, CMI, FAMI
Bill Andrews & Associates, Inc.
Post Office Box 300885
Medical Center Station
Houston, TX 77230-0885
(713) 668-8897

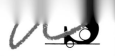

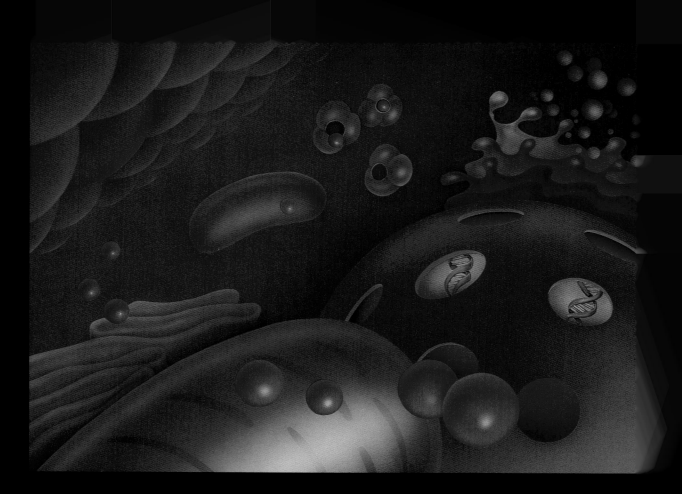

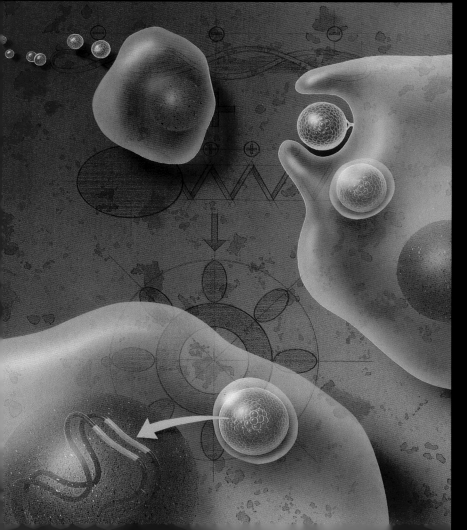

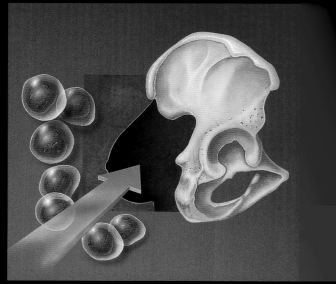

amy p. collins
samuel k. collins

art and science,® inc.
medical and graphic illustration

2815-A 18th Street South
Birmingham, AL 35209
(205) 871-4445
(205) 871-4465 fax

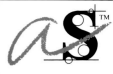

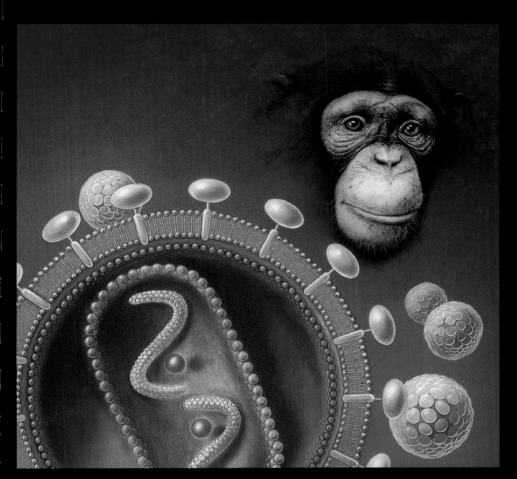

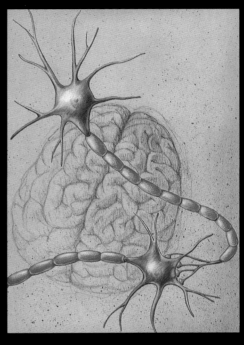

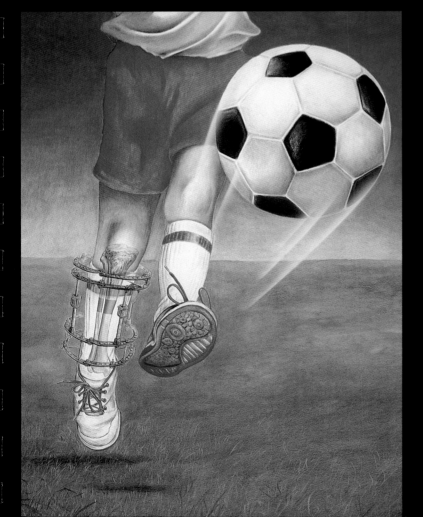

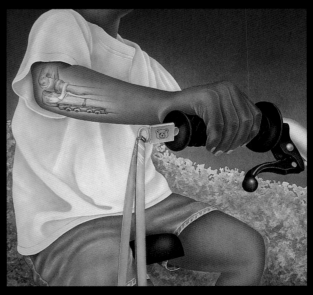

amy p. collins
samuel k. collins

art and science,® inc.
medical and graphic illustration

2815-A 18th Street South
Birmingham, AL 35209
(205) 871-4445
(205) 871-4465 fax

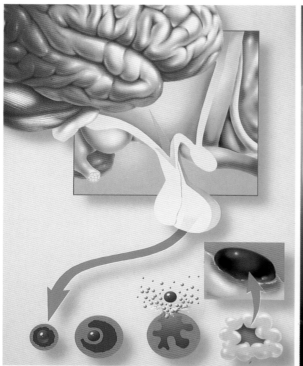

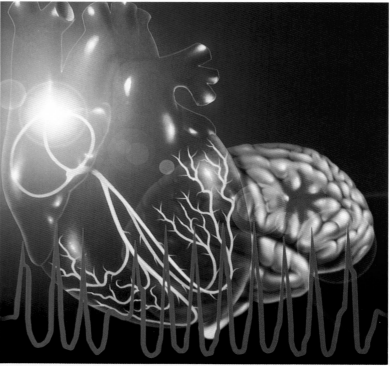

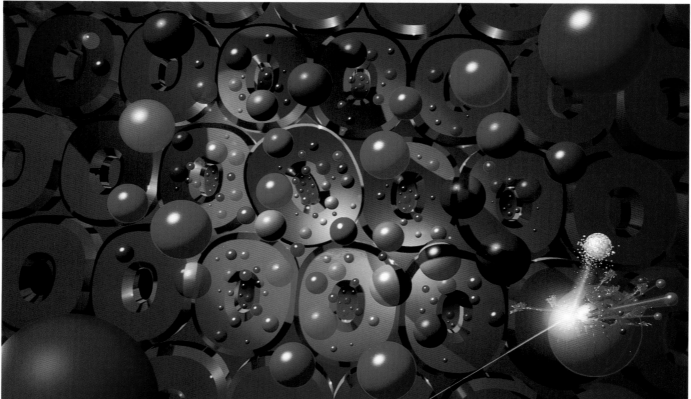

ALEXANDER & TURNER

Edmond Alexander, CMI
56 Old Miller Place
Grayton Beach, FL 32459
(904) 231-4112
FAX (904) 231-4142

Represented by **ARTCO** LLC
Serving New York City:
Gail Thurm and Tammy Shannon
232 Madison Avenue, Suite 402
New York, NY 10016
(212) 889-8777   FAX (212) 447-1475

Serving Clients outside New York City:
Jeff Palmer
227 Godfrey Road
Weston, CT 06883
(203) 222-8777   FAX (203) 454-9940

SPECIALIZATION
High impact illustration for publishers, pharmaceutical companies and their agencies has
long been the hallmark of art from Edmond
Alexander. His ability to synthesize complex
functions and mechanisms of the human body
and present them in a unique color and style
has resulted in three decades of award-winning
images.

IMAGES FOR REUSE
Alexander and Turner has hundreds of images
on numerous medical topics available for reuse.

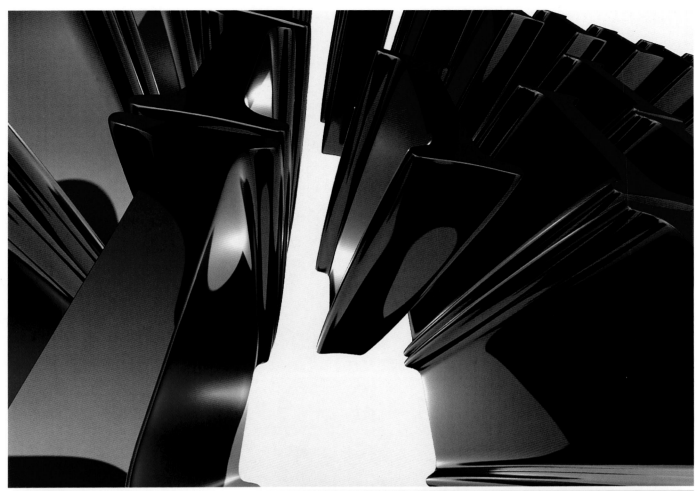

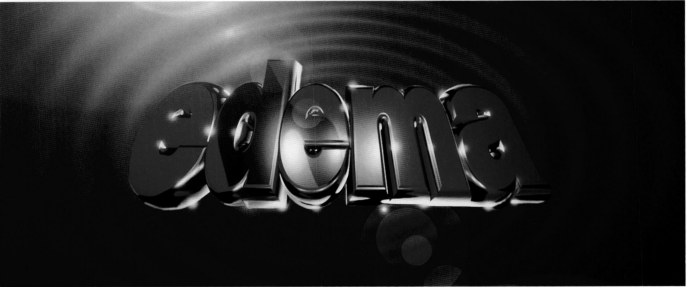

ALEXANDER & TURNER
Edmond Alexander, CMI
56 Old Miller Place
Grayton Beach, FL 32459
(904) 231-4112
FAX (904) 231-4142

DIGITAL ART
The one thing that will always separate the artist from the computer . . . is the artist. It is the artist's sensitive orchestration of design, color, composition and message that creates the successful work. The computer provides a sophisticated medium for obtaining the result.

MULTIMEDIA
The production of multimedia requires a fluent understanding of design, illlustration, graphics, text, photography, motion, sound, and animation. Edmond Alexander has demonstrated proficiency in each for almost three decades. He understands the power of an interactive media and recognizes the potential of electronic multimedia.

BOOK ART ON DISKS
Art samples from biology and medical texts are available on disks upon request.

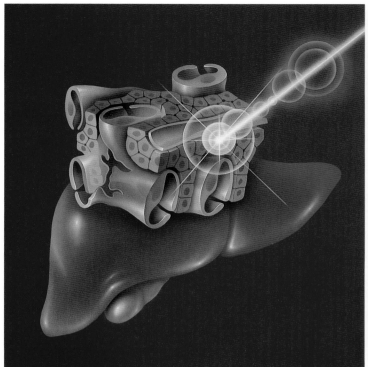
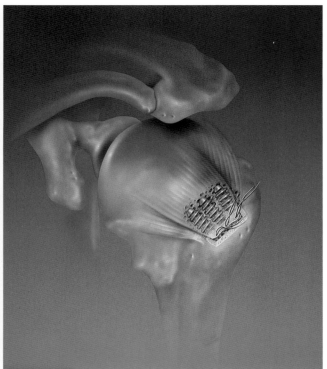
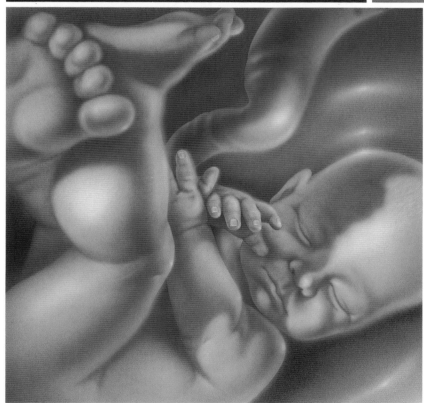
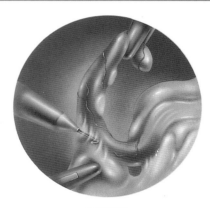
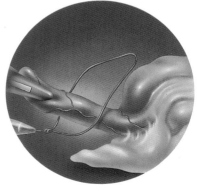

ALEXANDER & TURNER

Cynthia Turner, CMI
56 Old Miller Place
Grayton Beach, FL 32459
(904) 231-4112
FAX (904) 231-4142

Represented by **ARTCO** LLC
Serving New York City:
Gail Thurm and Tammy Shannon
232 Madison Avenue, Suite 402
New York, NY 10016
(212) 889-8777   FAX (212) 447-1475

Serving Clients outside New York City:
Jeff Palmer
227 Godfrey Road
Weston, CT 06883
(203) 222-8777   FAX (203) 454-9940

SPECIALIZATION

Visualizing the functions and mechanisms of the human body with color, depth, realism and academic content is the hallmark of art from Cynthia Turner. Her ability to place the viewer inside the body and provide answers beyond the questions has resulted in her recognition as one of the country's premier medical illustrators for pharmaceutical, product, editorial and textbook illustration.

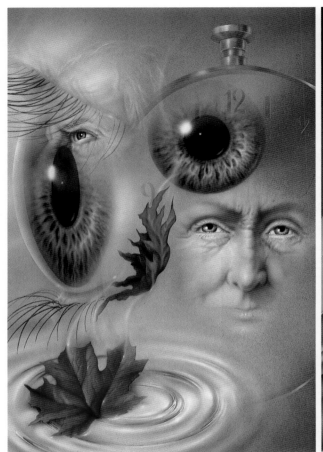
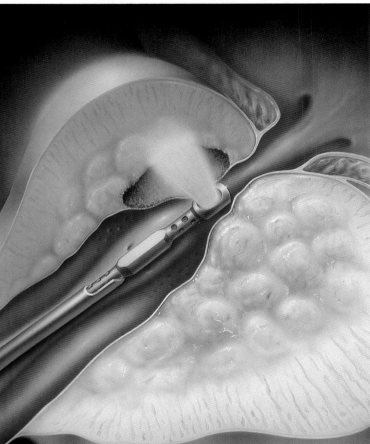
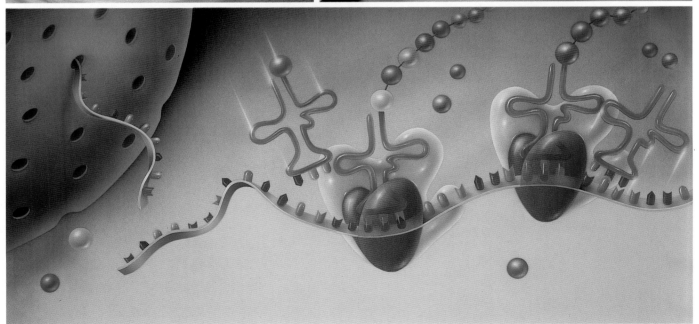

ALEXANDER & TURNER

Cynthia Turner, CMI
56 Old Miller Place
Grayton Beach, FL 32459
(904) 231-4112
FAX (904) 231-4142

ADVERTISING ILLUSTRATION

Illustrations for pharmaceutical and bio-technology subjects include mode-of-action, pathophysiology, physiological cascades and lyrical interpretations of drug action.

PRODUCT ILLUSTRATION

Highlighting attributes of medical products and instrumentation includes showcasing the product interacting in its environment.

EDITORIAL ILLUSTRATION

Often recognized for the enormous scope of the subjects she paints, Cynthia continues to seek painting assignments that provide challenges and expand her horizons.

TEXTBOOK ILLUSTRATION

Simplicity of presentation and sophistication of execution appropriately describe Cynthia's approach to textbook art.

ARTCO

STUDIO MACBETH

Digital Illustration, Retouching, Photography, Electric Image Manipulation

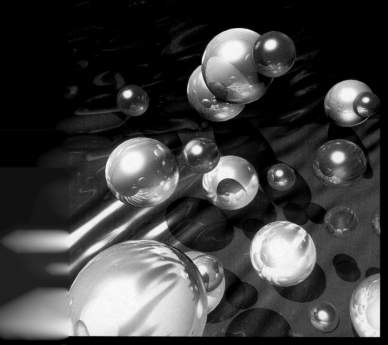

Drug Attached to White Corpuscle

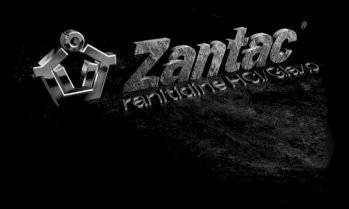

3D Model of Marble and Gold Logo

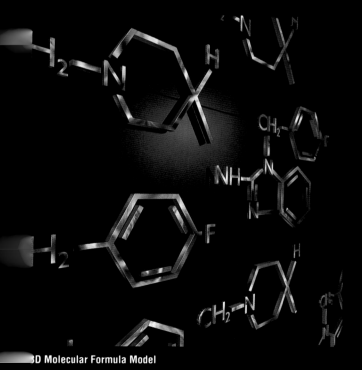

3D Molecular Formula Model

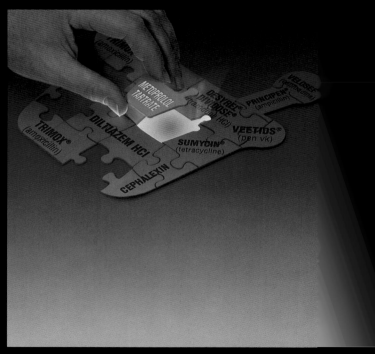

Photo Montage Plus Special Effects

ARTCO L.L.C. • Gail Thurm and Jeff Palmer • Tammy Shannon, Associate

clients within New York City: 232 Madison Avenue • Room 402 • New York, NY 10016   (212) 889-8777 • Fax: (212) 44

clients outside New York City: 227 Godfrey Road • Weston, CT 06883   (203) 222-8777 • Fax: (203) 45

STUDIO MACBETH

Digital Illustration, Retouching, Photography, Electric Image Manipulation

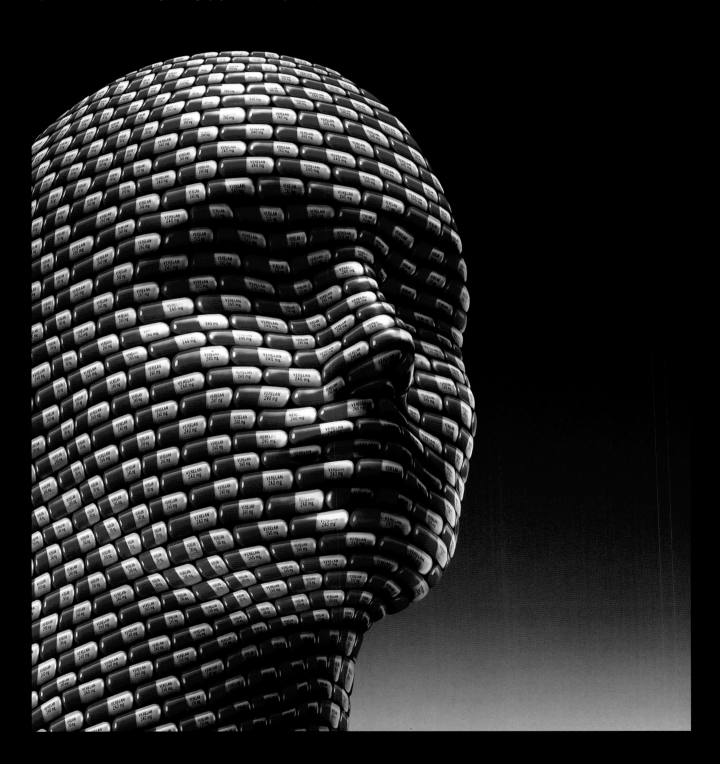

ARTCO L.L.C. • Gail Thurm and Jeff Palmer • Tammy Shannon, Associate

Serving clients within New York City: 232 Madison Avenue • Room 402 • New York, NY 10016   (212) 889-8777 • Fax: (212) 447-1475
Serving clients outside New York City: 227 Godfrey Road • Weston, CT 06883   (203) 222-8777 • Fax: (203) 454-9940

DOUG STRUTHERS

Computer Illustration, Animation

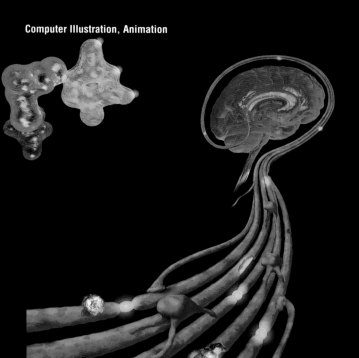

The Processes of Multiple Sclerosis

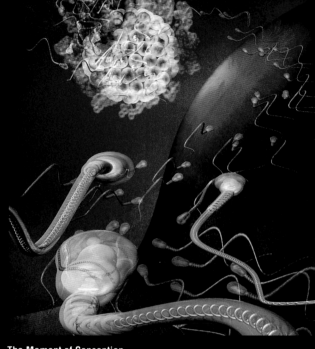

The Moment of Conception

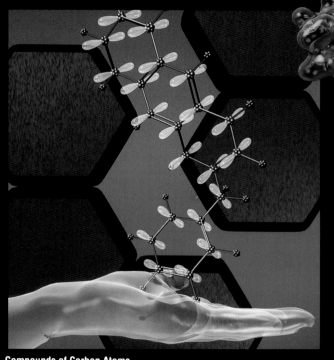

Compounds of Carbon Atoms

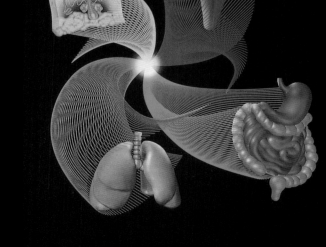

Zosyn

ARTCO L.L.C. • Gail Thurm and Jeff Palmer • Tammy Shannon, Associate

Serving clients within New York City: 232 Madison Avenue • Room 402 • New York, NY 10016   (212) 889-8777 • Fax: (212) 447-1475
Serving clients outside New York City: 227 Godfrey Road • Weston, CT 06883   (203) 222-8777 • Fax: (203) 454-9940

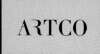

DOUG STRUTHERS

Computer Illustration, Animation

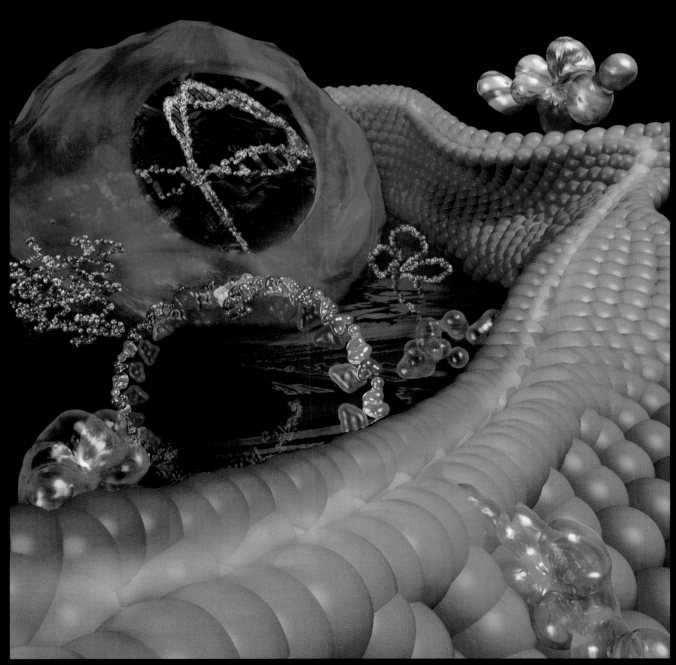

Cell. Nucleus. Protein. and Nucleic Acid

ARTCO L.L.C. • Gail Thurm and Jeff Palmer • Tammy Shannon, Associate

Serving clients within New York City: 232 Madison Avenue • Room 402 • New York, NY 10016   (212) 889-8777 • Fax: (212) 447-1475
Serving clients outside New York City: 227 Godfrey Road • Weston, CT 06883   (203) 222-8777 • Fax: (203) 454-9940

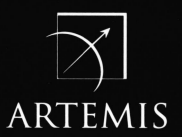

ARTEMIS

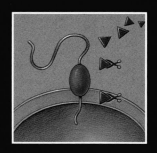

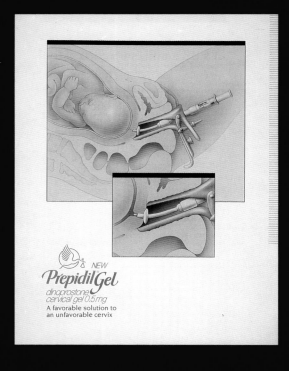

NEW
Prepidil Gel
dinoprostone
cervical gel 0.5mg
A favorable solution to
an unfavorable cervix

Artemis is an illustration and design studio dedicated to the clear and creative communication of complex scientific ideas. We take great pride in our work for pharmaceutical, biotechnology, and high technology companies, healthcare institutions, attorneys, and publishers. We work directly with our clients or their public relations and advertising agencies.

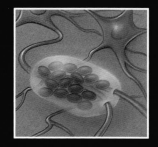

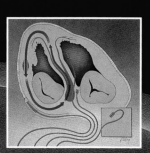

Our clients include Addison-Wesley, Alza, Applied Biosystems, Athena Neurosciences, Becton Dickinson, Intel Corporation, Medical Economics, Mitsubishi Electronics, Syntex Laboratories, and The Upjohn Company.

Our work has won a Gold award from the Medical Marketing Association and four First Place awards from the Association of Medical Illustrators.

Betsy A. Palay, M.S., FAMI
Certified Medical Illustrator

721 Emerson Street
Palo Alto, CA 94301
Phone (415) 325-6596
Fax (415) 325-0446

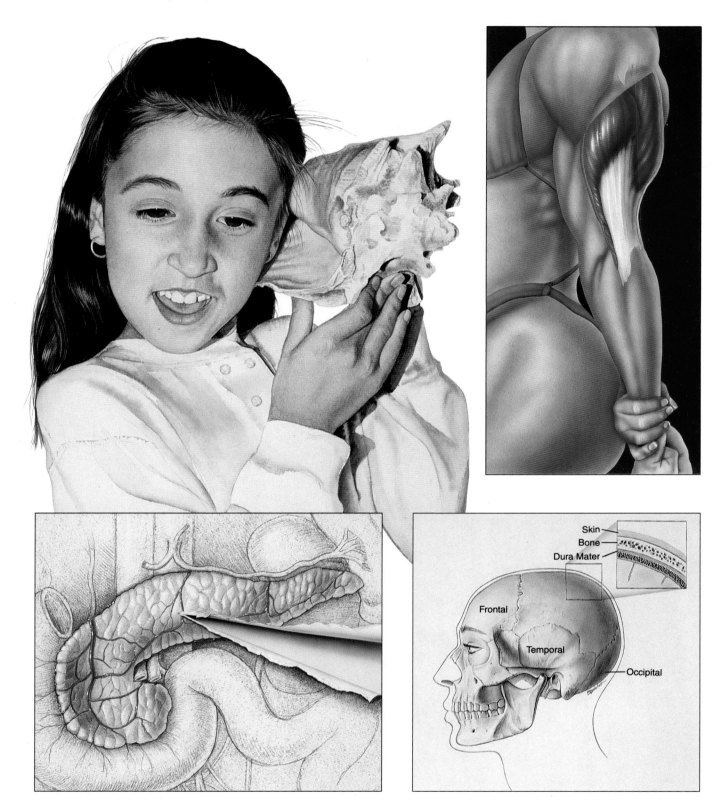

MOLLY BABICH
413 Wabash Street
Fort Collins, Colorado 80526
(303) 223-1779

AREAS OF SPECIALIZATION: Anatomical, surgical, biological illustrations for textbooks, journals and commercial applications. Special interests in patient education and health and fitness information.

PROFESSIONAL BACKGROUND: M.S., Anatomy/Biomedical Illustration, Colorado State University. Five years full-time freelance illustration. AMI member.

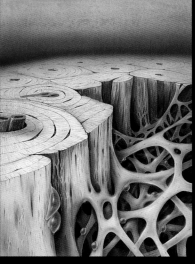
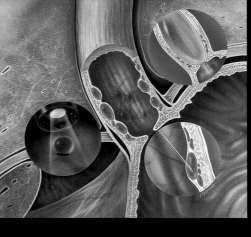
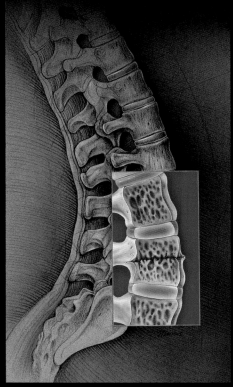
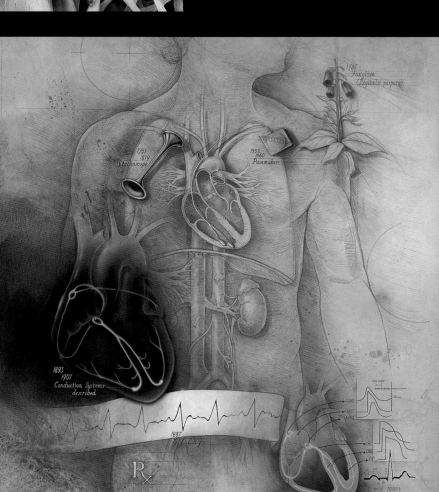
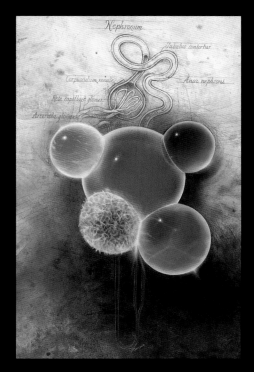

SCOTT THORN BARROWS
Medical Art Associates
5182 Cypress-on-Ohio St.
Lisle, IL 60532
(708) 969-6263   FAX (708) 969-6298

AREAS OF SPECIALIZATION: All forms of medical illustration, including creative development for video, animation, virtual reality, museum displays, and computer-generated art. Extensive medical background and clinical consultant base.

PROFESSIONAL BACKGROUND: Clinical Assistant Professor, University of Illinois at Chicago Medical Center. Former Medical Art Director at ad agency and Assistant Professor at University of Texas Southwestern Medical Center. Honors graduate, University of Illinois Medical Center. Outstanding Alumnus Award, UIC.

PROFESSIONAL MEMBERSHIPS: CMI, FAMI, Association of Medical Illustrators; Alumni Board, College of Associated Health Professions, UIC.

CLIENTS: Advertising agencies, pharmaceutical companies, medical instrumentation, publishers, museums, hospitals, and foundations.

AWARDS/HONORS: Numerous national and international awards. Artwork in National Library of Medicine Archives, Smithsonian, Chicago Museum of Science and Industry, Nobel Conferences, and select collections.

OTHER: Portfolio available. Many illustrations available for re-use. Studio Macintosh Quadra-based.

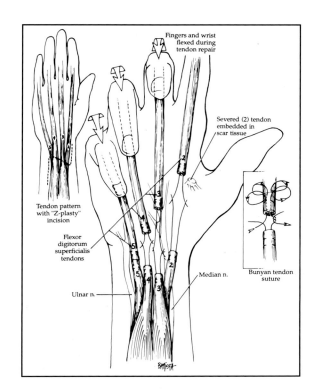

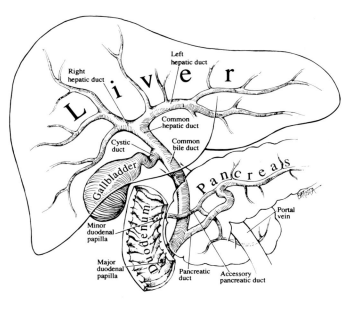

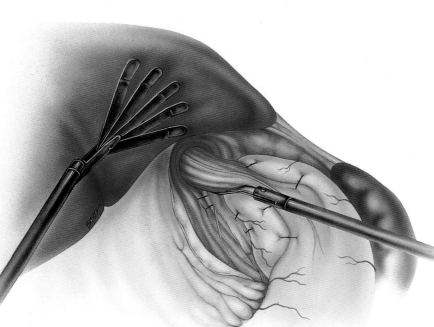

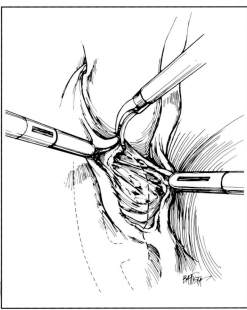

KIMBERLY M. BATTISTA
1307 Hollins Street
Baltimore, Maryland 21223
Phone/FAX (410) 685-7988

SPECIALIZATION: Currently illustrating for text book & journal publishers, major medical product manufacturers, and multimedia presentations (computer and video). Expertise in surgical illustration; specialization in current laparoscopic procedural illustration.

BACKGROUND: Received a Master of Arts degree from The Johns Hopkins University School of Medicine.

CLIENTS: U.S. Surgical Corporation, Williams & Wilkins, Mosby Yearbook, Multimedia Presentation Systems Inc., private surgeons, physicians, and attorneys.

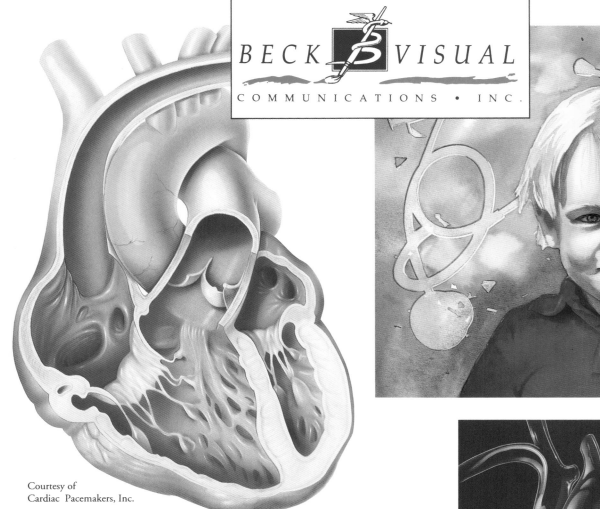

BECK B VISUAL
COMMUNICATIONS • INC.

Courtesy of
Cardiac Pacemakers, Inc.

Our specialties:
Medical-product promotion
Pharmaceutical advertising
Medical-legal exhibits
Editorial art
Textbooks

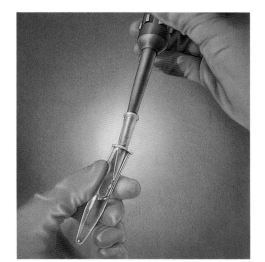

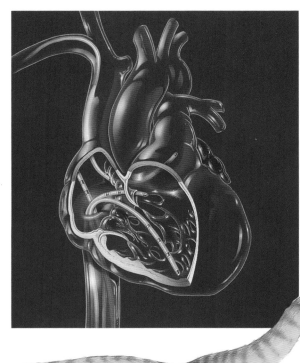

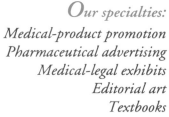

Outstanding service • On time • Within budget.
For more information, please contact:

Joan M. Beck, M.A., Certified

2525 E. Franklin Ave., Suite 201
Minneapolis, Minnesota 55406
Phone: (612) 338-8642
Fax: (612) 333-4438

Re-use:
Illustrations on a variety of subjects
and media are available for re-use.

Biomedia Corporation

is a full-service biomedical communication firm with a staff of talented medical illustrators, sculptors, and animators who create visual solutions for the health care industry.

Biomedia approaches each project on an individual basis after analyzing the subject matter, client requirements, cost factors and target audience. We consult with you to develop the concept, select the content, and produce an original product.

Biomedia has designed and produced award-winning

anatomical models

and

computer animations

for product promotion, patient education, continuing medical education, consumer information and litigation.

Our clients include:

Abbott Laboratories ❖ Robert A. Clifford & Associates ❖ Corboy and Demetrio ❖ Glaxo, Incorporated ❖ Lavey/Wolff/Swift, Incorporated ❖ Eli Lilly & Company ❖ Marion Laboratories ❖ Merck, Sharp & Dohme ❖ Pfizer Laboratories ❖ G.D. Searle & Company ❖ Schering Laboratories ❖ Sieber & McIntyre ❖ E. R. Squibb & Sons, Inc.

Diane L. Nelson, Certified Medical Illustrator
President
Master of Health Professions Education
Member and Fellow, Association of
   Medical Illustrators
Past chair, AMI Board of Governors
Clinical Assistant Professor, University of Illinois,
   Department of Biomedical Visualization
Winner of numerous awards from
   the Rx Club of New York, the AMI,
   the Institute of Graphic Arts,
   and the Biocommunications Forum

Please call

708/501-5560

for a demo tape
or samples
and receive a free
anatomical gift.
Ask for Diane.

SCOTT BODELL

9617 VINEWOOD DRIVE

DALLAS, TEXAS 75228

TELEPHONE:

214•648•9046

OR

214•320•3354

FACSIMILE:

214•648•7603

OR

214•320•8433

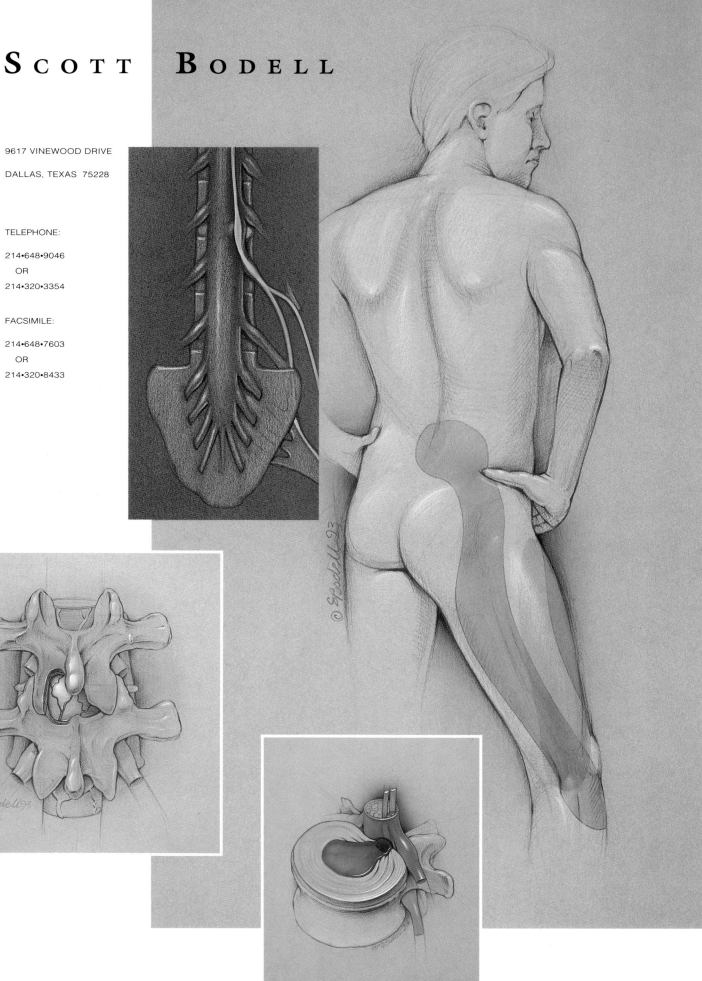

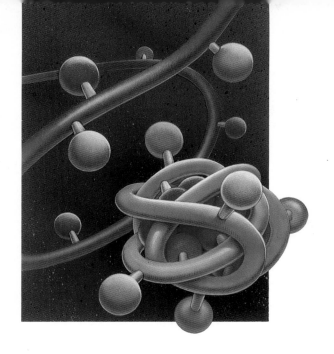

BIOMEDICAL IMAGERY FOR EDUCATIONAL,

ADVERTISING AND EDITORIAL PUBLICATION.

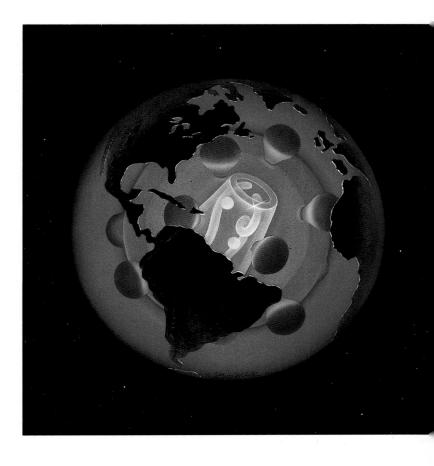

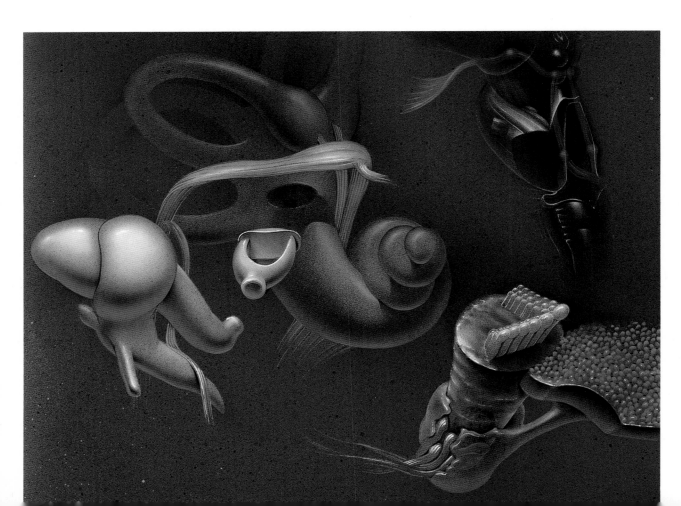

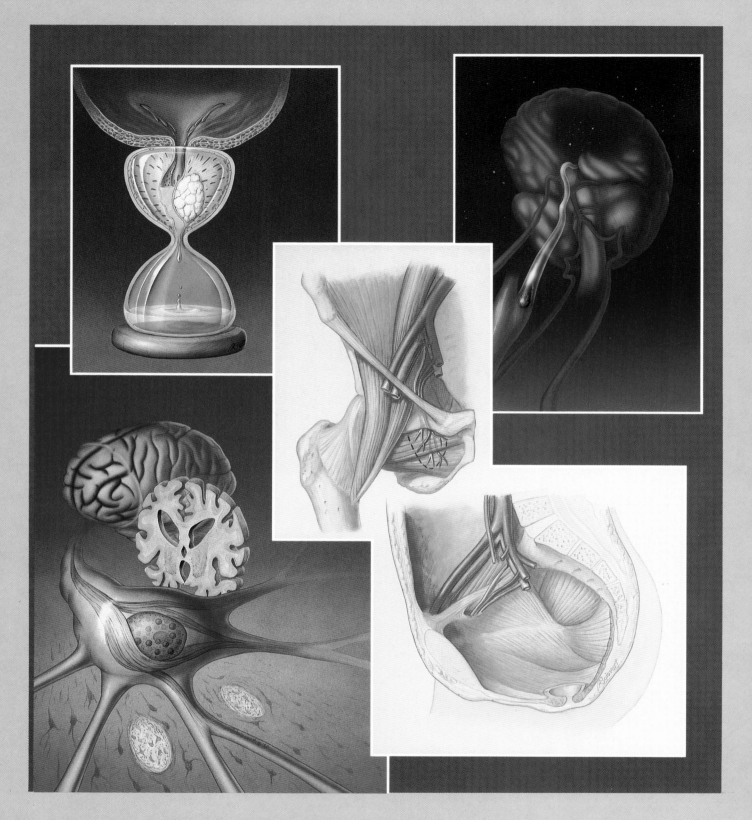

Ron Boisvert, MS, CMI

RGB Medical *Imagery*

162 E. Dunedin Rd.
Columbus, OH 43214
(614) 784-9918, 268-7719

AREAS OF SPECIALIZATION: Visual problem solving for the medical and health science professions. Surgical, anatomical, and conceptual illustration depicting human form and function. Specializing in orthopaedics and sports medicine.

PROFESSIONAL MEMBERSHIPS: Association of Medical Illustrators.

CLIENTS: Various publishing companies, medical journals, advertising agencies, medical products companies, health care institutions, and attorneys.

PROFESSIONAL BACKGROUND: Undergraduate degree in biology from the University of Connecticut. M.S. degree in Medical Illustration from the Medical College of Georgia, '83.

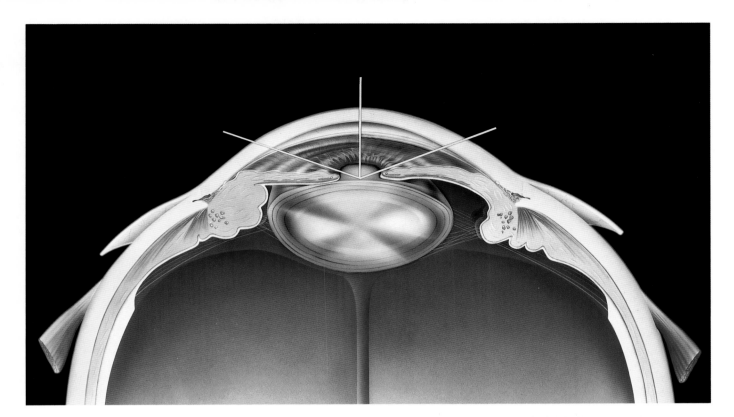

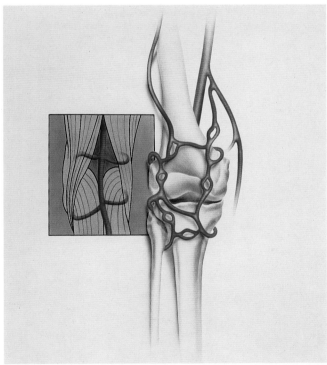

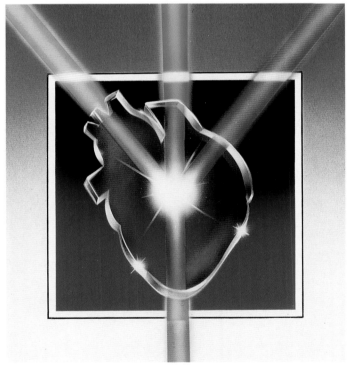

CLAIRE BOOTH MEDICAL ILLUSTRATION, AMI   2 WEST 46TH STREET,   NEW YORK, NY 10036   212-768-1829

L. CLAIRE BOOTH
Claire Booth Medical Illustration
2 West 46th Street
c/o Zazula Assoc., 2nd Fl.
New York, NY 10036
(212) 768-1829

PROFESSIONAL BACKGROUND: BFA, BS, Georgia College, Milledgeville, GA. Graduate studies: Johns Hopkins Medical Institute, Dept. of Art as Applied to Medicine, MA Medical Illustration program.

PROFESSIONAL MEMBERSHIPS: Association of Medical Illustrators.

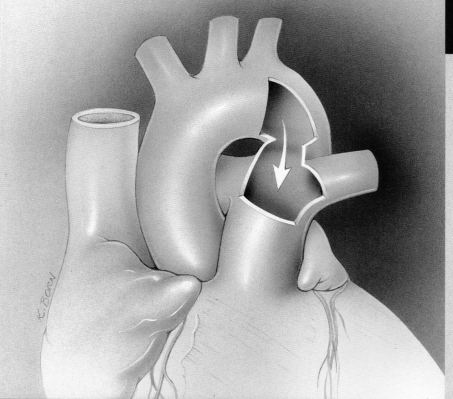

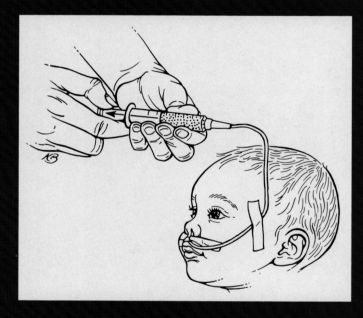

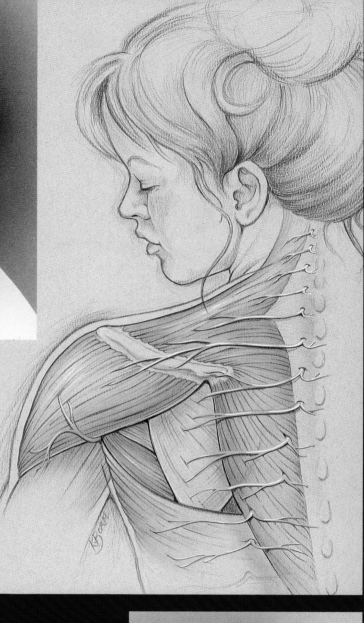

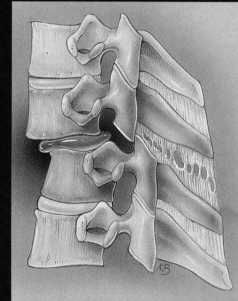

KATHRYN BORN, M.A.
Certified Medical Illustrator
P.O. Box 200663
Arlington, TX 76006
Phone/FAX Metro (817) 640-7052

PROFESSIONAL BACKGROUND: M.A. in medical illustration, Univeristy of Texas. B.A. in Fine Arts/Biology, College of William and Mary. Former staff illustrator, Johns Hopkins. Currently self-employed.

AWARDS/HONORS: AMI Salon judge, 1993; Rx Club, NY, Award of Excellence, 1992; AMI Medical Book Award, 1988.

PUBLICATIONS: Artwork appears in *Operative Techniques in Orthopedics* (W.B. Saunders); *Patient Care Magazine* (Medical Economics); *Current Therapy in Sports* (Mosby-Year Book); *Advances in Trauma and Critical Care* (Cooper Hospital); *The Care of the Pediatric Nasogastric Tube* (Cooper Hospital); *Rehabilitation of the Spine* (Springer-Verlag); *A Textbook of Transesophageal Echocardiography* (Elsevier); and numerous *American Academy of Family Physicians* publications.

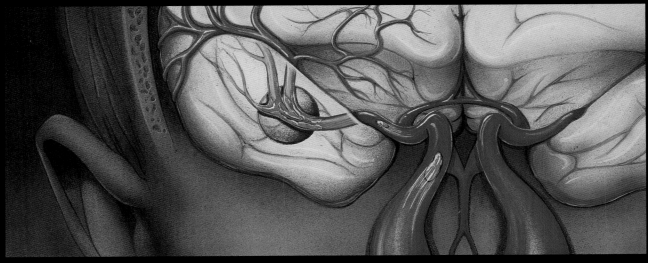

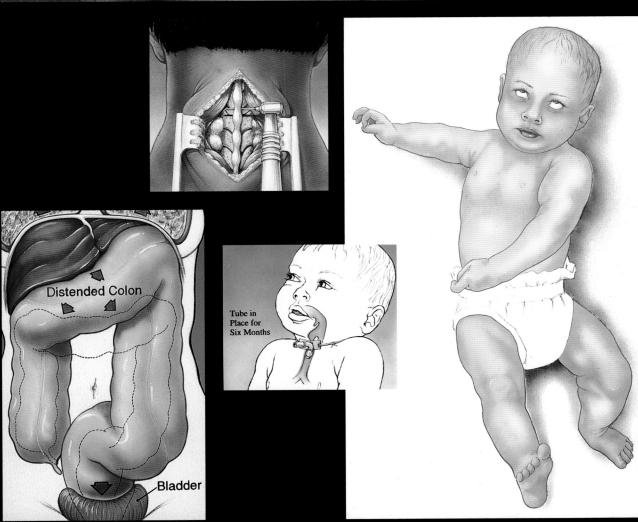

Distended Colon

Bladder

Tube in
Place for
Six Months

ELLEN BOYLAN
E. B. Studio
8831 Antrim Avenue
Dallas, TX 75218
(214) 320-4947

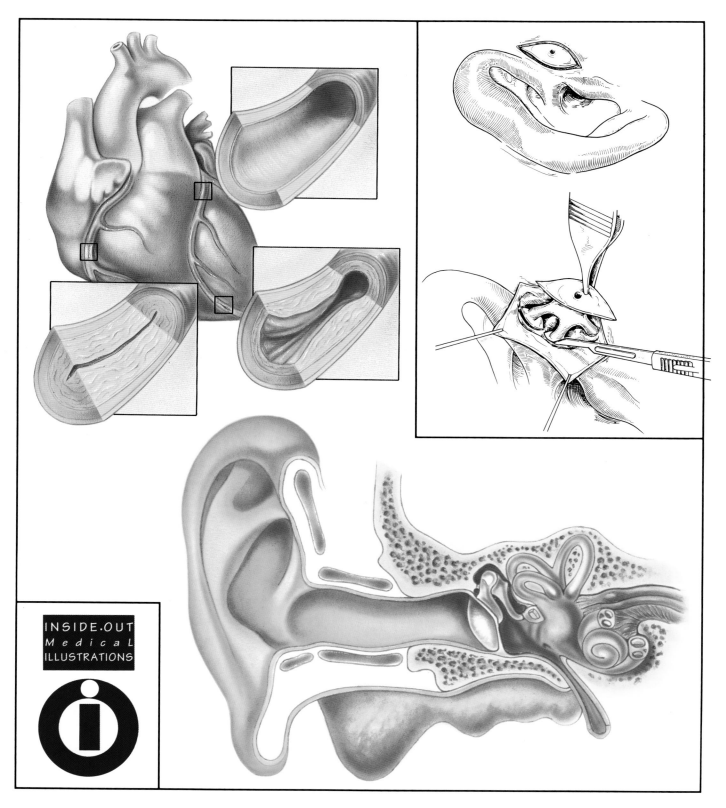

SUSAN SHAPIRO BRENMAN
Inside-Out Medical Illustrations
33 Great Neck Road, Suite 11
Great Neck, NY 11021
(516) 466-8658
FAX (516) 466-4048

AREAS OF SPECIALIZATION: Full color medical and surgical illustration for advertising, editorial, and medical-legal markets. Continuous tone and line illustrations for patient education and text publications.

PROFESSIONAL BACKGROUND: M.S. Medical Illustration, University of Rochester School of Medicine and Dentistry.

PROFESSIONAL MEMBERSHIPS: Association of Medical Illustrators, Guild of Natural Science Illustrators.

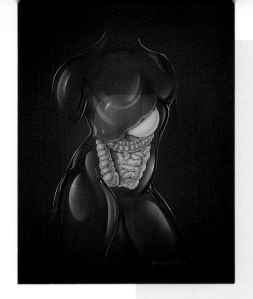

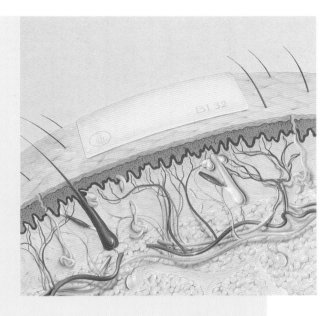

BRYSON

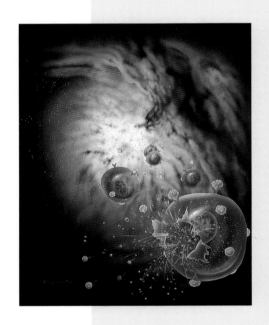

Mary K. Bryson, M.A.M.S., C.M.I.

Bryson Biomedical Illustrations
2401 Pennsylvania Avenue
Suite 605
Wilmington, DE 19806

Telephone: (302) 888-1134
Fax: (302) 888-1243

Professional Background

Master of Associated Medical Science,
Biomedical Visualization,
University of Illinois at Chicago.
Bachelor of Fine Arts, Graphic
Design, Washington University.
Certified Medical Illustrator

Client List Available Upon Request

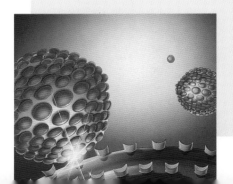

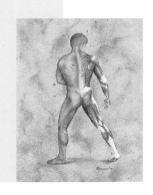

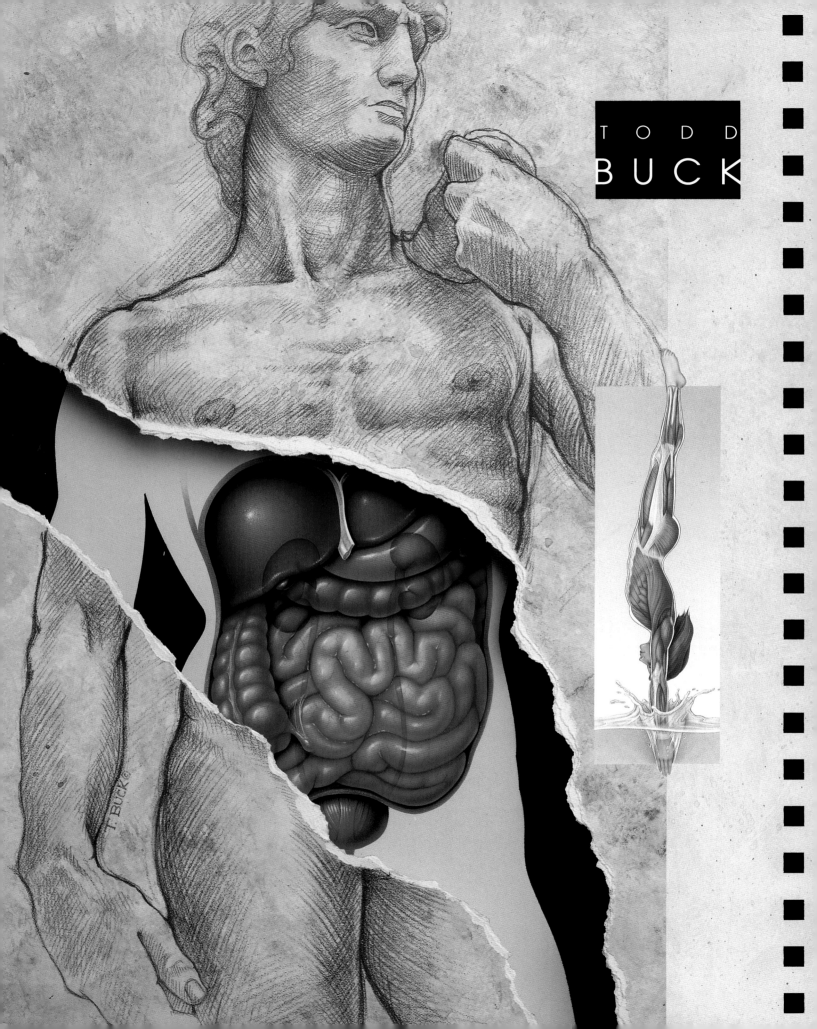

TODD BUCK

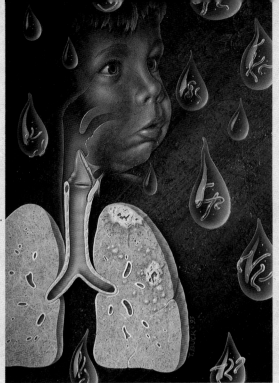

medical
illustration

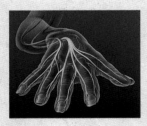

TODD BUCK

3 Elizabeth Court
Lombard, Illinois
60148

Telephone
and Fax
Number
(708) 627■0903

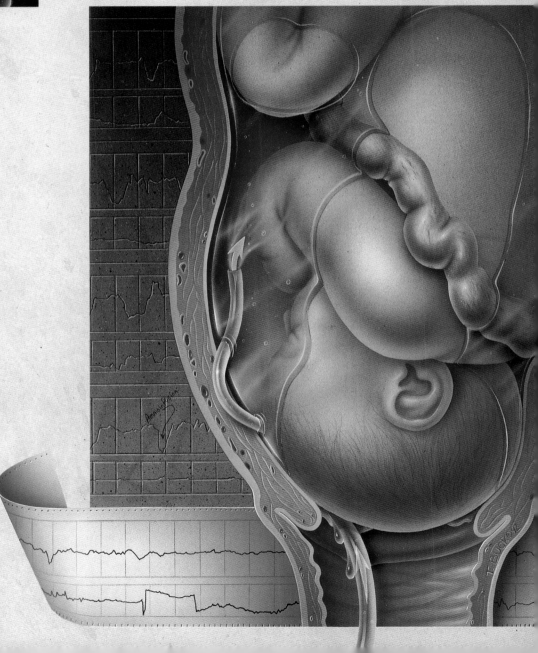

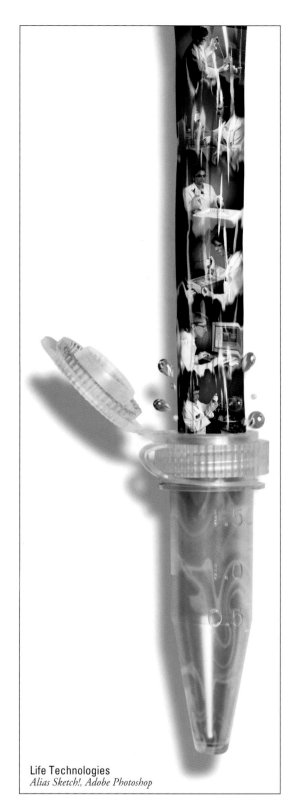

Life Technologies
Alias Sketch!, Adobe Photoshop

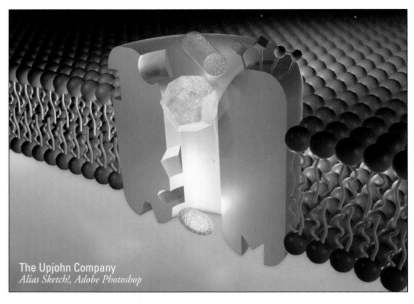

The Upjohn Company
Alias Sketch!, Adobe Photoshop

The Appropriate Solutions

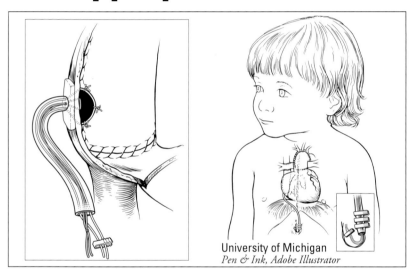

University of Michigan
Pen & Ink, Adobe Illustrator

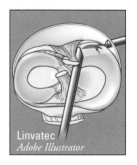

Linvatec
Adobe Illustrator

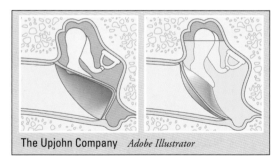

The Upjohn Company   *Adobe Illustrator*

Innovation and sophistication are the appropriate solutions for your scientific and medical illustration needs. Experience includes art production for print and projection media and animation for video and multimedia CDs. Silver award recipient in the Rx Club Show of Medical Advertising.

Christopher Burke

4408 Chad Court   *voice:* **313-996-1316**

Ann Arbor, Michigan   *fax:* **313-996-5820**

48103-9478   *modem:* **313-996-5801**

A certified member of the Association of Medical Illustrators and adjunct assistant professor at the University of Michigan School of Art.

All copyrights and product names are property of their respective holders.

·C·A·L·D·E·R·

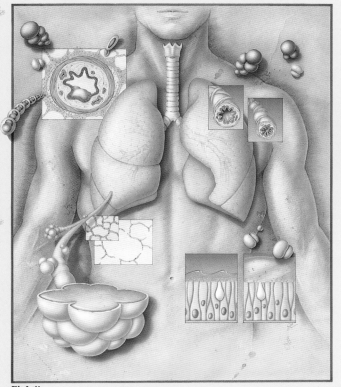

Eli Lilly

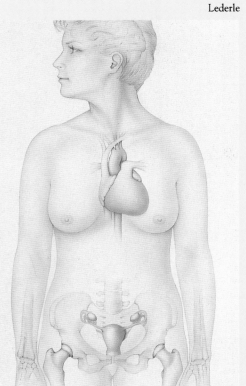

Lederle

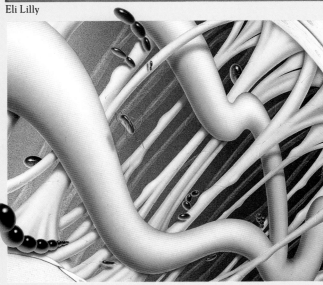

Editorial: Bacteria

Ciba-Geigy: Menopause

· MEDICAL ILLUSTRATION ·

Jean E. Calder B.A., B.Sc. AAM

New York (212) 808-0018   Toronto (416) 484-6349

Margie Caldwell-Gill

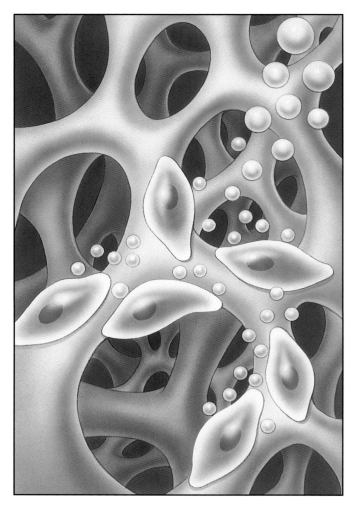

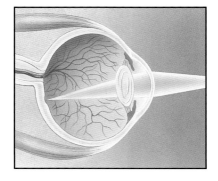

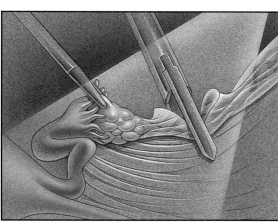

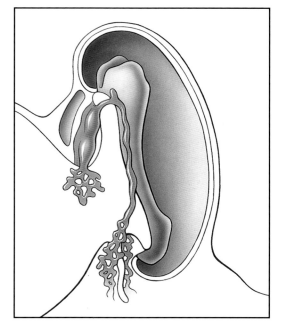

MARGIE CALDWELL-GILL, C.M.I.
105 Abbeywood Drive
Nashville, TN 37215
Phone/FAX (615) 665-9188

AREAS OF SPECIALIZATION: Clear communication of complex anatomical concepts for: Advertising, PR and Collateral materials; Editorial support; Patient education materials; Medical-legal exhibits.

CLIENTS: Medical and pharmaceutical advertising agencies; publishers of medical and scientific journals and textbooks; medical schools and hospitals; private physicians and attorneys.

PROFESSIONAL BACKGROUND: M.A., Medical Illustration, The University of Texas Southwestern Medical Center, 1987. Active Member of the Association of Medical Illustrators since 1989. Certified Medical Illustrator.

AWARDS: Association of Medical Illustrators Annual Salon: First Place for Reference Text, 1993; First Place for Medical Color, 1992; Second Place for Medical Color, 1990.

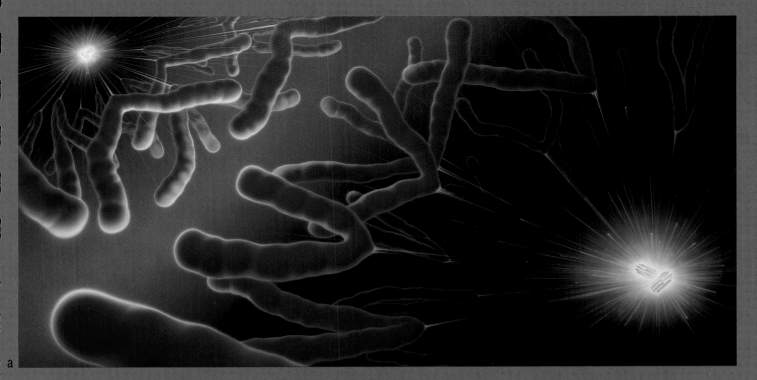
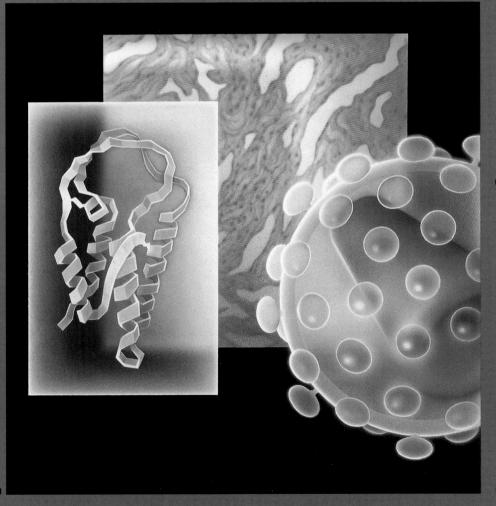
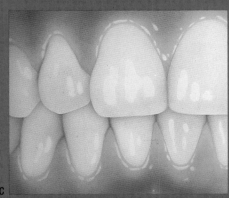
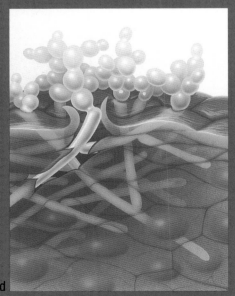

a

b

c

d

GARY CARLSON

ILLUSTRATION

BIOLOGICAL & MEDICAL

25 Kinnicutt Road East Pound Ridge, NY 10576
914·764·5828 Phone & Fax

a. Cell mitosis in anaphase.
b. Sarcoma, alpha interferon, AIDS virus.
c. Healthy and pearly.
d. Candida, firmly entrenched.

May S. Cheney Medical and Scientific Illustration

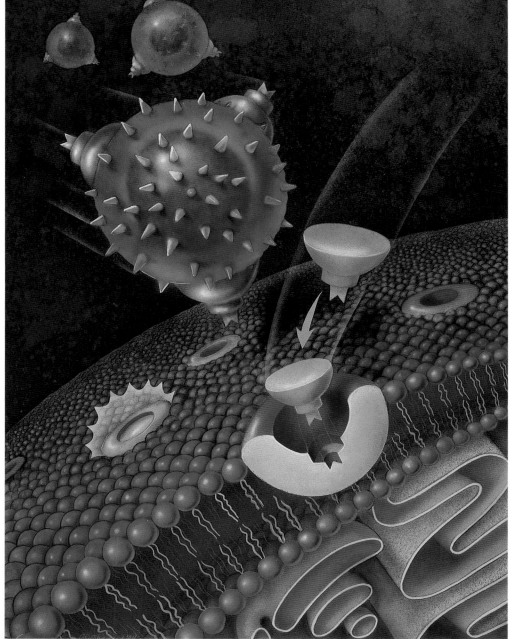

Anatomical & conceptual medical illustration in color, line, or tone. Communication for patient education, journal publications, educational texts and research technologies.

6220 N. 14th Place Phoenix, Arizona 85014

TEL (602) 279-2840

FAX (602) 266-4175

Professional Background: BA, UCLA; MA, University of Texas Southwestern Medical School. Certified Medical Illustrator.

Professional Memberships: AMI, GNSI.

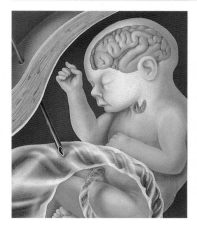

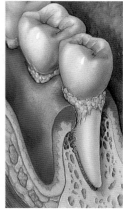

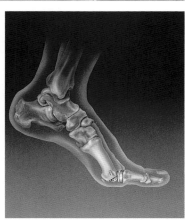

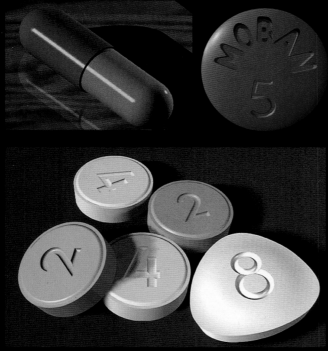
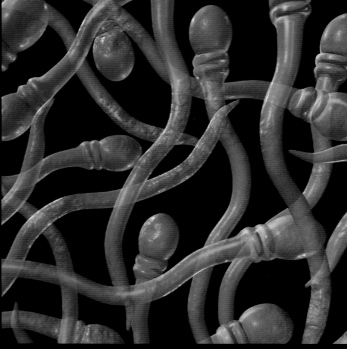
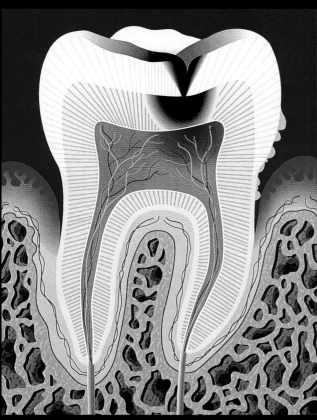
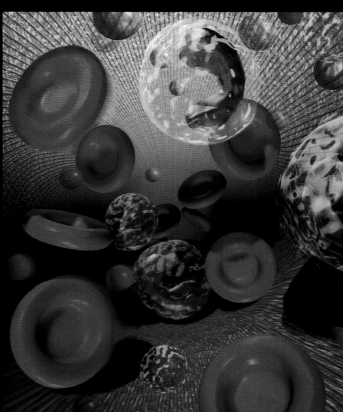

ANATOLY CHERNISHOV

4 Willow Bank Court
Mahwah, NJ 07430-2909
(201) 327-2377
FAX/Modem (201) 236-9469

AREAS OF SPECIALIZATION:
Medical & Pharmaceutical illustration
Advertising & product promotion
Editorial, poster & book illustration
Full color & B/W illustration
Airbrush & computer illustration.

CLIENTS: Block Drug Co., Blunt-Hann-Sersen,
Carrafiello-Diehl, Dugan/Farley, Ferguson Communications Group, Sterling Health, Lavey/
Wolff/Swift, Kallir, Philips, Ross, Medical Economics, Sudler & Hennessey.

PROFESSIONAL MEMBERSHIPS:
Association of Medical Illustrators.

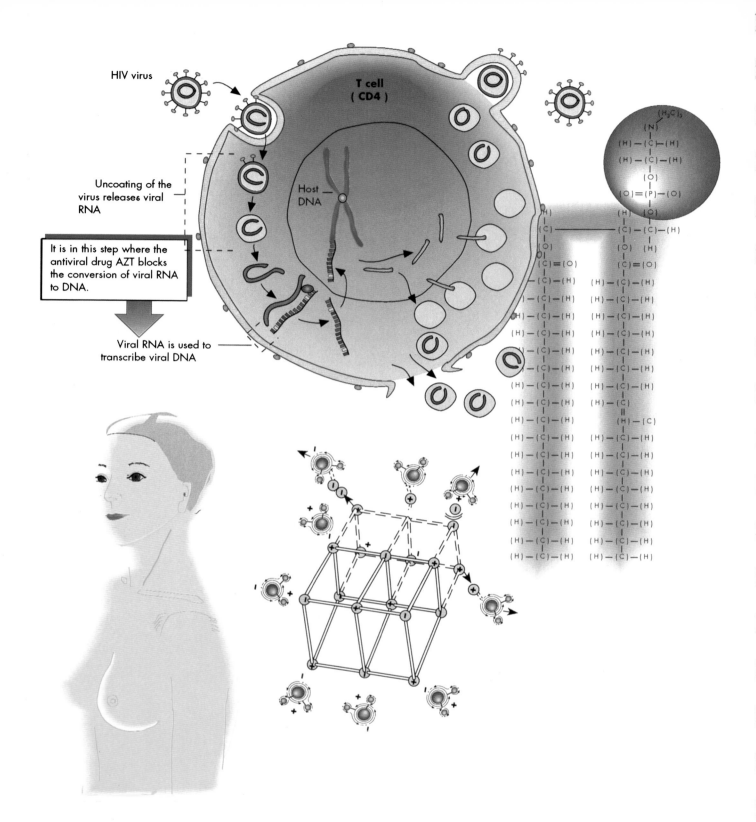

HIV virus

T cell
(CD4)

Uncoating of the
virus releases viral
RNA

Host
DNA

It is in this step where the
antiviral drug AZT blocks
the conversion of viral RNA
to DNA.

Viral RNA is used to
transcribe viral DNA

THEODATE COATES
433 West Broadway
New York, NY 10012
(212) 966-7292

AREAS OF SPECIALIZATION:
Biochemistry illustration—
cells
cancer
viruses
heredity
cholesterol

MEDIUM:
Computer

PROFESSIONAL MEMBERSHIPS:
AMI

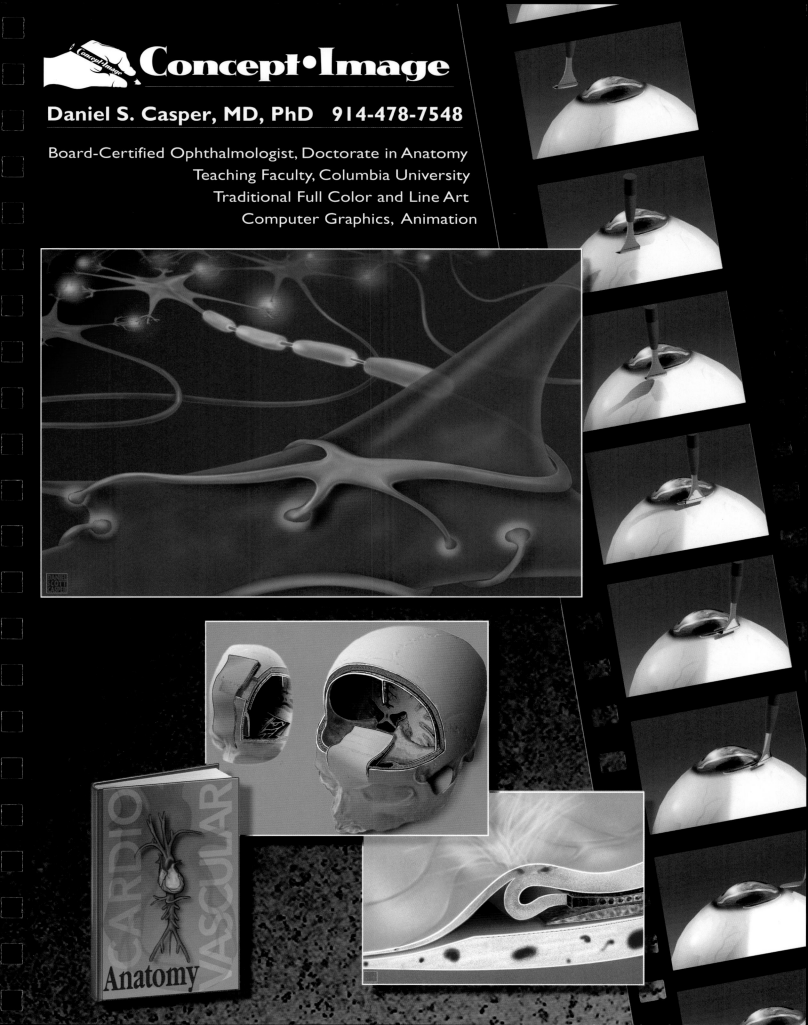

Concept•Image

Daniel S. Casper, MD, PhD   914-478-7548

Board-Certified Ophthalmologist, Doctorate in Anatomy
Teaching Faculty, Columbia University
Traditional Full Color and Line Art
Computer Graphics, Animation

CARDIO VASCULAR Anatomy

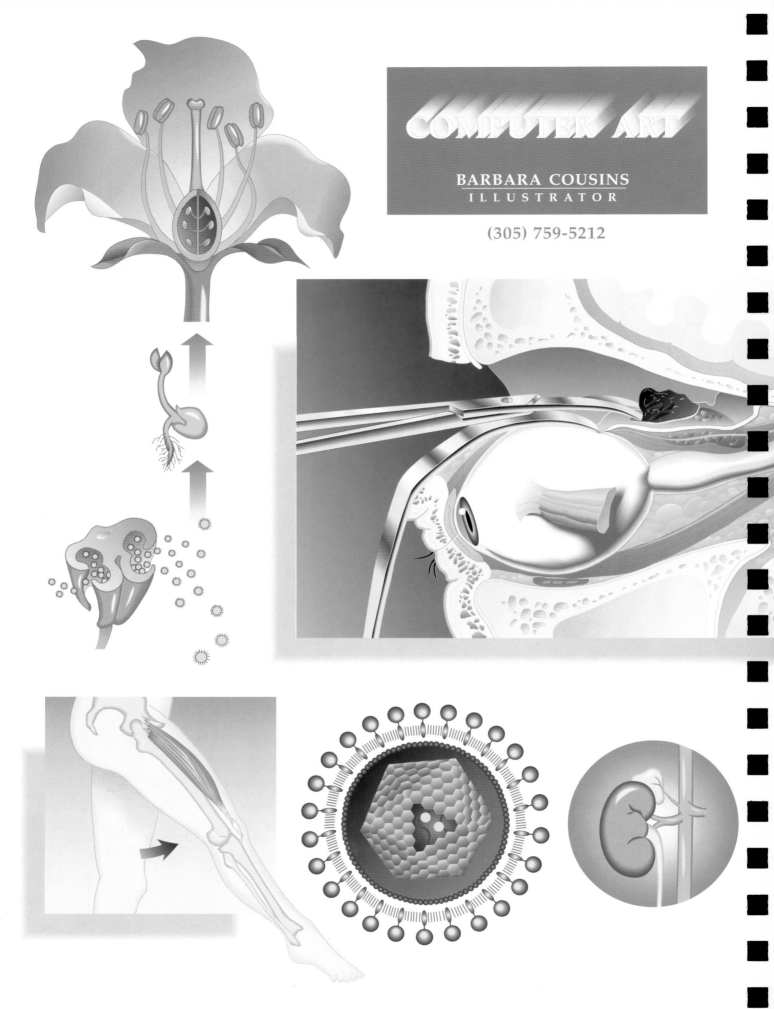

COMPUTER ART

BARBARA COUSINS
ILLUSTRATOR

(305) 759-5212

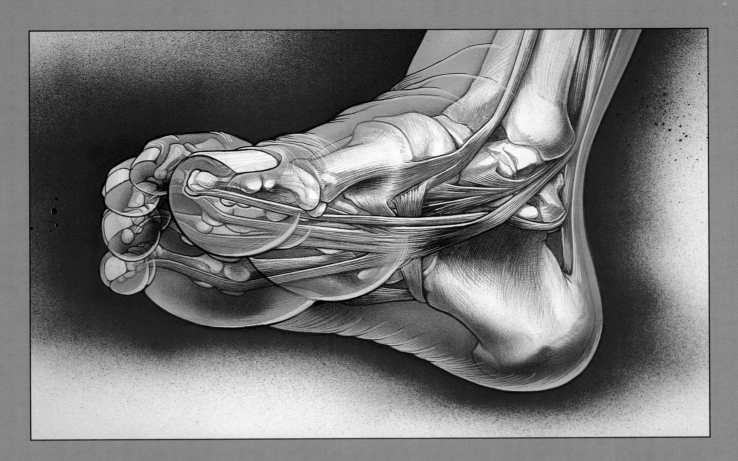

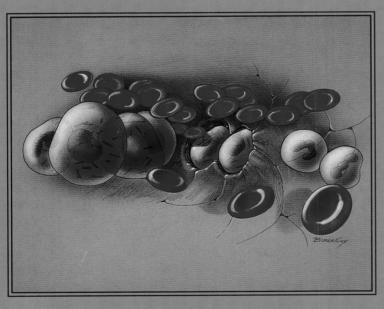

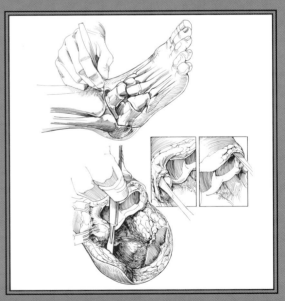

BIRCK COX

Birck Cox Medical Illustration
514 E. Allens Lane
Philadelphia, PA 19119
(215) 242-5102 H, W, F

AREAS OF SPECIALIZATION: Orthopedics, Artificial Organs, Cardiac Surgery, Cell Ultrastructure.

CLIENTS: A.H. Robins Pharmaceuticals, Arrow International, Interspec Ultrasound Inc., *Diagnosis* Magazine, *Geriatrics* Magazine, Micro-Straight, Inc., *Nursing 94* Magazine, Anatomical Chart Co., Saunders College Publishing, Williams & Wilkins/Harwal Publishing.

PROFESSIONAL BACKGROUND: B.A. English, Reed College; M.S. Med. Ill. Medical College of Georgia, 1980; Texas Tech University, Lubbock; Medical College of Virginia, Richmond; Hershey Medical Center (Penn State University), Hershey; Fulltime Freelance in Southeastern PA.

PROFESSIONAL MEMBERSHIPS:
Certified, Association of Medical Illustrators.

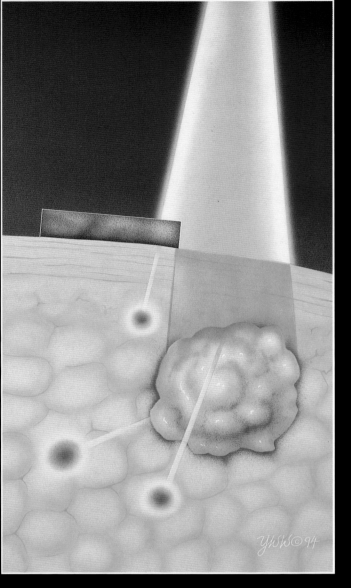

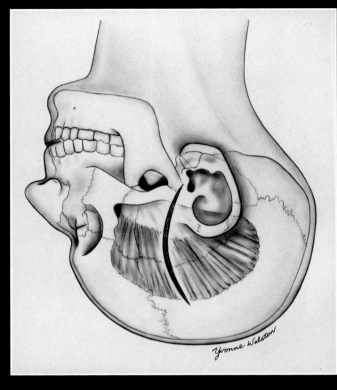

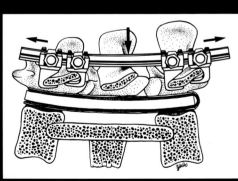

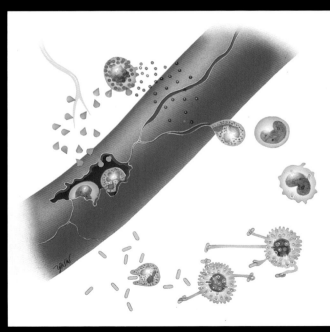

CREATIVE IMAGERY, INC.

Yvonne W. Walston, MA, CMI
3640 High Street, N.E.
Albuquerque, NM 87107
Phone/FAX (505) 344-8986

AREAS OF SPECIALIZATION: Full-service visual communications studio, with award-winning, problem-solving artists. Computer graphics and animations as well as traditional techniques of line, tone and color illustration raphy. Graphic design. 3D models. Includes forensic exhibits.

PROFESSIONAL BACKGROUND: *Education:* M.A. in Medical Illustration, the University of Texas Southwestern Medical Center. B.S. in Zoology, University of Kentucky. *Experience:* Over thirteen years in medical illustration, including six years at UNM Biomedical Communications. Four years as medical researcher.

PROFESSIONAL MEMBERSHIPS: Association of Medical Illustrators, Rio Grande SIGGRAPH.

AWARDS: From the Association of Medical Illustrators and the Society for Technical Communication.

All projects receive the same competent attention and creative consideration. We are here to make your successful communication on time

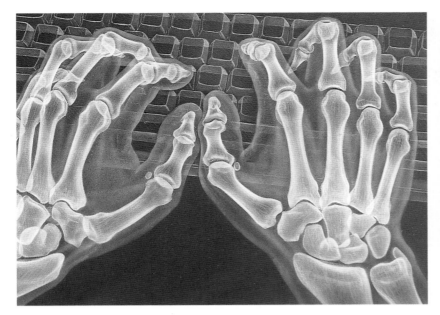

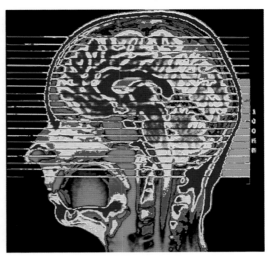

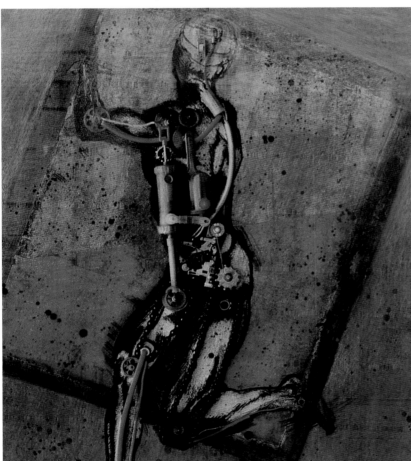

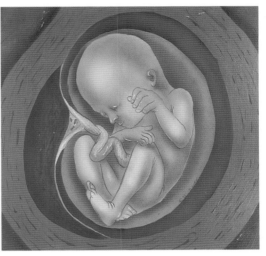

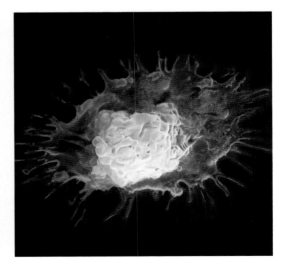

**CUSTOM MEDICAL
STOCK PHOTO, INC.**
3819 North Southport Avenue
Chicago, IL 60613-2823
(800) 373-2677
(312) 248-3200
FAX (312) 248-7427

AREAS OF SPECIALIZATION: Custom Medical Stock Photo specializes in stock photography and illustration created by the most talented medical artists and medical photographers in the world.

CLIENTS: Custom Medical Stock Photo's clients include publishers and advertising agencies worldwide. Available from CMSP are the stock catalog *The Medical Book, Volume One* and *The Medical Book, Volume One Photo CD*.

PROFESSIONAL MEMBERSHIPS: PACA, ASPP, BPA.

Clockwise from top left: Hands on Keyboard by Todd Buck, MRI by R. Porter, 22 week fetus by Delilah Cohn, SEM of a single Breast Cancer Cell by AMC, How the Body Moves by Marc Galindo. All rights reserved, copyright Custom Medical Stock Photo 1995.

MARIE DAUENHEIMER

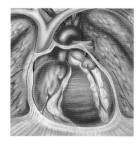

Marie T. Dauenheimer
Medical Illustration Studio
11808 Breton Court
Suite 22B
Reston, Virginia 22091
(703) 648-9038 Phone/FAX
In New York City:
(718) 463-2607

Specializing in surgical, anatomical and conceptual illustration for books, magazines, patient education, advertising and video.

Animation services
include storyboards, 2D and 3D animation using Macintosh and Silicon Graphics. Video demo reel available upon request.

Professional background includes M.A. in Medical Illustration from the Johns Hopkins School of Medicine. Board Certified Medical Illustrator. Experience as Art Director for medical video production company.

Awards/Honors:
Association of Medical Illustrators, Certificate of Merit in Animation, 1990 and 1993.

3D images featured here were created at Fast Cuts Video, Washington, DC

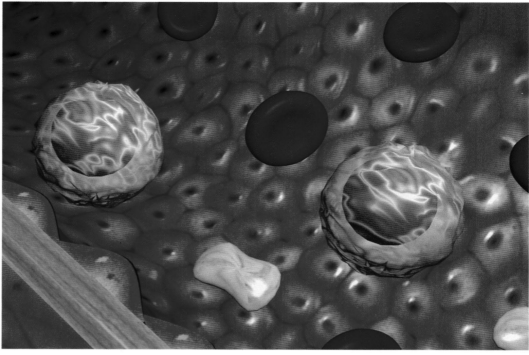

Copyright 1993 American College of Cardiology

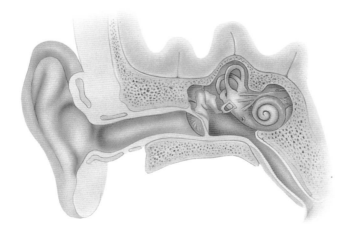

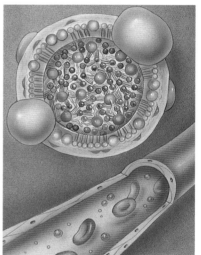

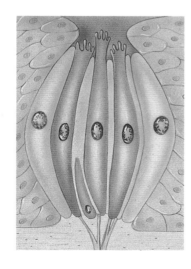

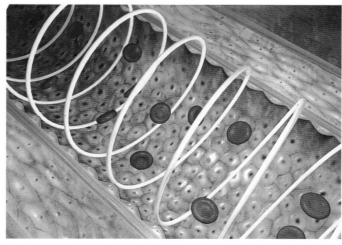

Copyright 1993 American College of Cardiology

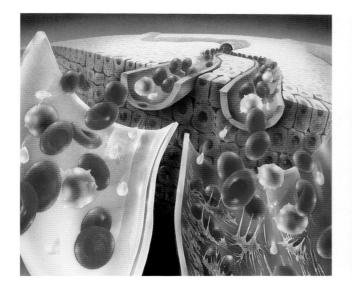

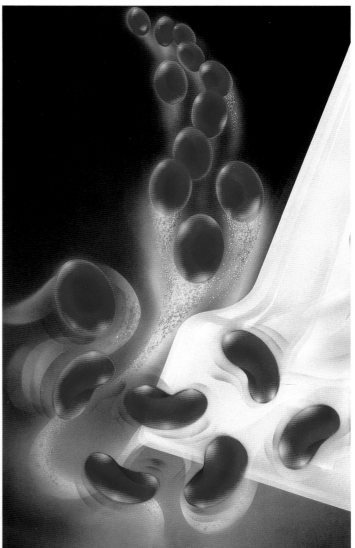

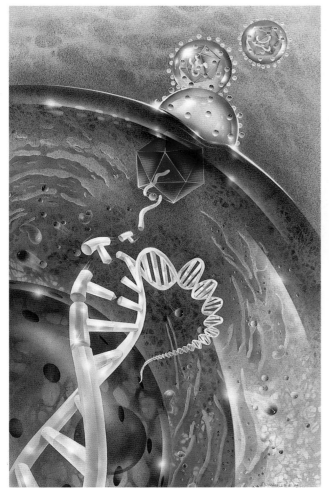

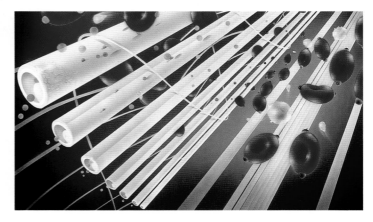

JIM DOWDALLS

12750 E. Centralia St. #128
Lakewood, CA 90715
(310) 865-9550
FAX (310) 860-6221

AREAS OF SPECIALIZATION: Full color medical and conceptual illustration for editorial, advertising, and exhibit presentation.

CLIENTS: Amgen, Inc., Baxter Healthcare, Inc., Upjohn, Inc., Johnson and Johnson, Inc., Ioptex Research, Inc., Medical Economics Publishing, Harcourt Brace Jovanovich, Journal of the American Medical Association, *Postgraduate Medicine* Magazine.

PROFESSIONAL BACKGROUND:

BFA, MA, Medical Illustration.

PROFESSIONAL MEMBERSHIPS:

Association of Medical Illustrators, Society of Illustrators, Los Angeles.

AWARDS/HONORS: Bronze Medal, Illustration West, 1993; Awards of Excellence (2), Rx Club, New York, 1992; Silver Medal, Illustration West, 1992; DESI Award of Excellence, Graphic Design USA, 1991; Honorable Mention, AMI Salon, 1990.

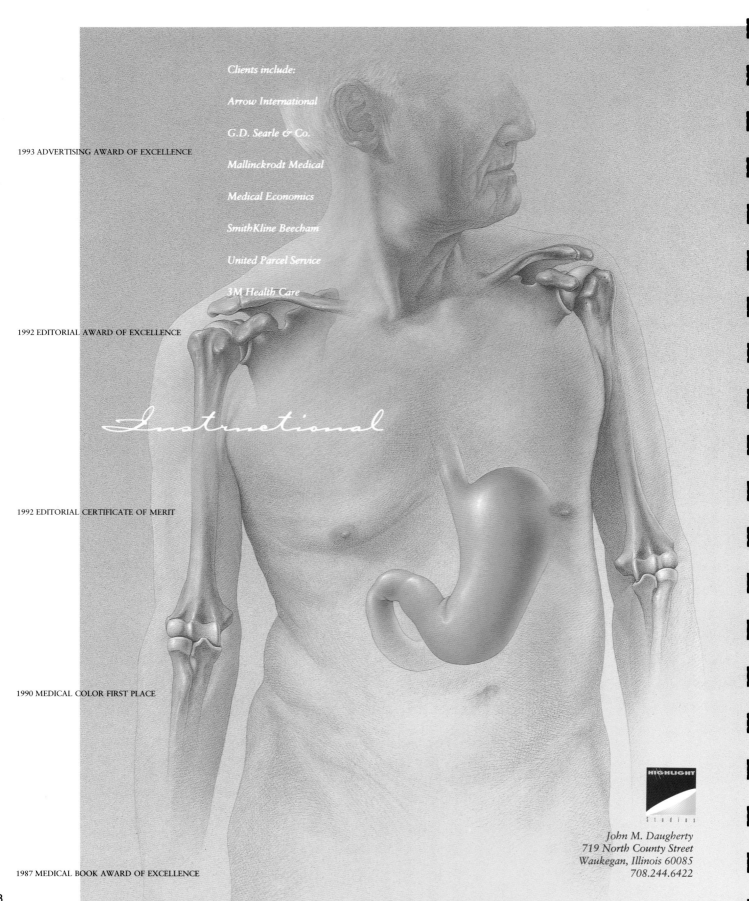

Promotional

Clients include:

Arrow International

G.D. Searle & Co.

Mallinckrodt Medical

Medical Economics

SmithKline Beecham

United Parcel Service

3M Health Care

1993 ADVERTISING AWARD OF EXCELLENCE

1992 EDITORIAL AWARD OF EXCELLENCE

Instructional

1992 EDITORIAL CERTIFICATE OF MERIT

1990 MEDICAL COLOR FIRST PLACE

1987 MEDICAL BOOK AWARD OF EXCELLENCE

HIGHLIGHT Studios

John M. Daugherty
719 North County Street
Waukegan, Illinois 60085
708.244.6422

Master of Science in Medical and Biological Illustration from

the University of Michigan. Board Certified. Currently, Clinical

Assistant Professor, Department of Biomedical Visualization,

The University of Illinois at Chicago.

Editorial

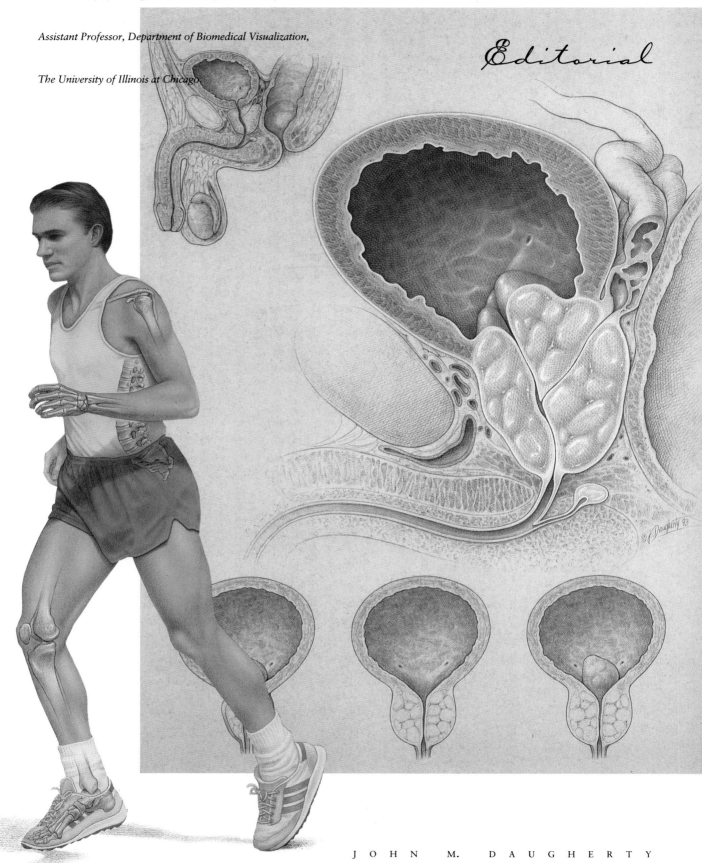

J O H N   M .   D A U G H E R T Y

CAROL
DONNER

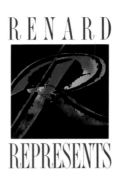

212-490-2450
FAX: 697-6828
EDITORIAL:
602-299-7107
FAX: 299-7670

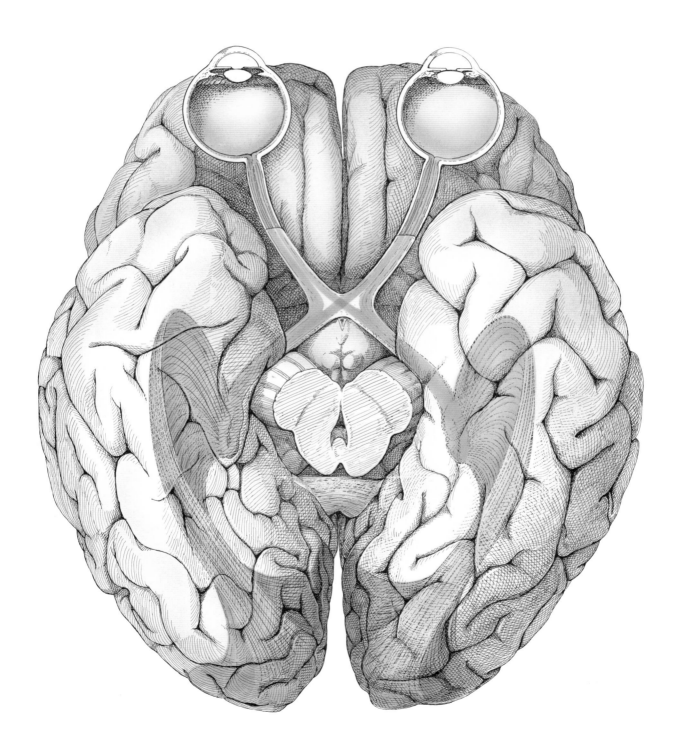

CAROL DONNER

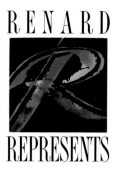

RENARD

REPRESENTS

212-490-2450
FAX: 697-6828
EDITORIAL:
602-299-7107
FAX: 299-7670

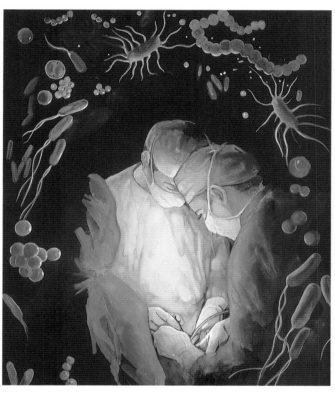

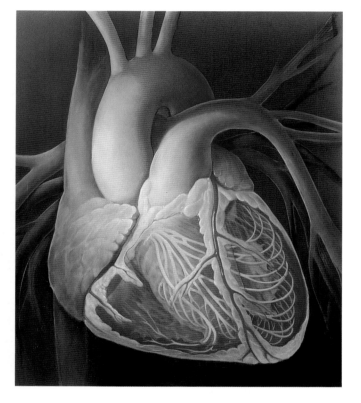

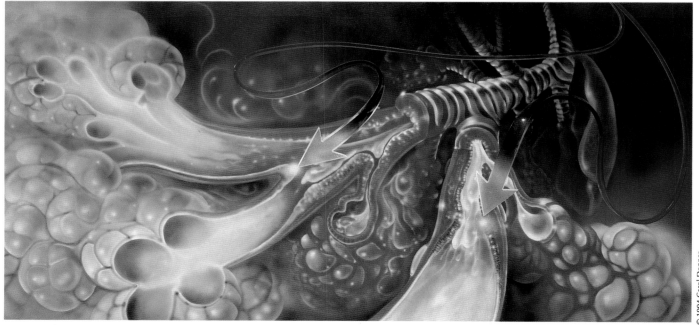

© 1994 Carol Donner

©American Electromedics

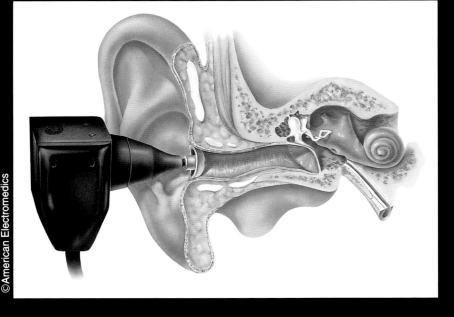

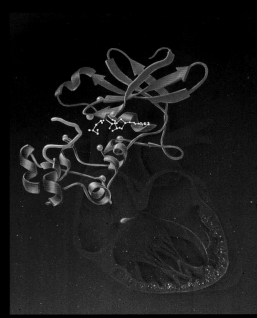

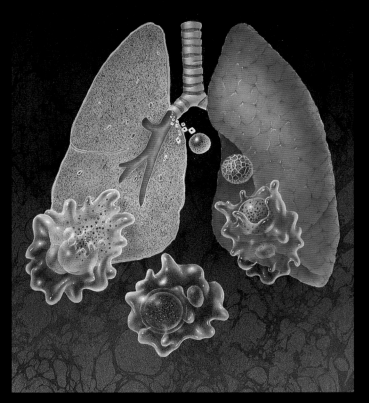

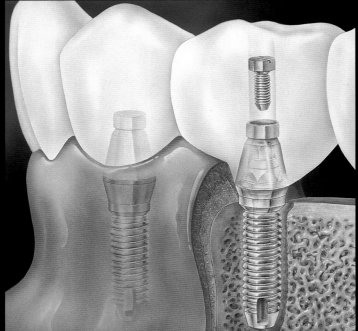

MEL DRISKO

Drisko Illustrations, Inc.   **234 Newport St. Denver, CO 80220**   **Tel/Fax: 303-399-4373**

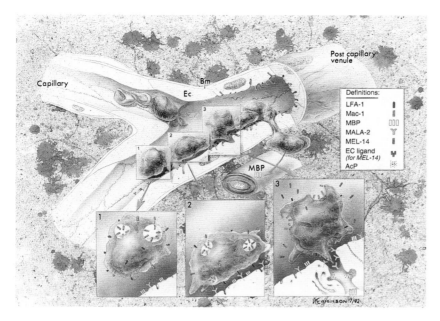

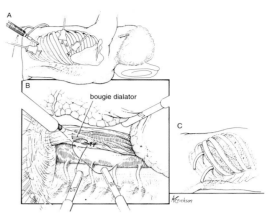

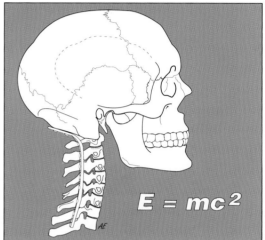

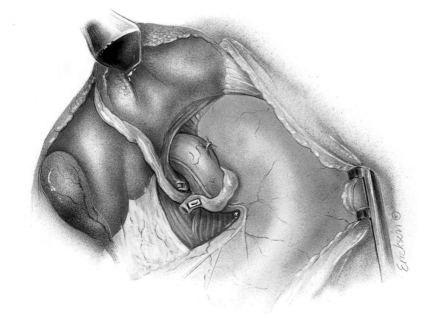

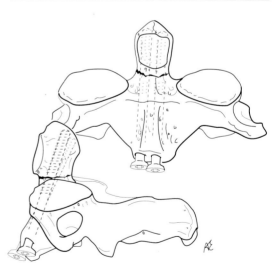

ANNE ERICKSON

E=mc² (Erickson = medical communications concepts)
78 Serrell Ave.
Staten Island, New York 10312
(718) 356-7705

AREAS OF SPECIALIZATION: Full color medical illustration, black & white (computer-generated and traditional line art) to the surgical, research and legal communities.

PROFESSIONAL BACKGROUND: B.S., Wagner College; 3 years Illustration/graphic design, Pratt Institute; M.A., Medical Illustration, Johns Hopkins. Freelance experience 1983–present.

CLIENTS: *Readers Digest*, Ortho Diagnostics, Veterans Affairs Medical Centers, Harwal Press, surgeons in metropolitan area and eastern Pennsylvania.

PROFESSIONAL MEMBERSHIPS: Association of Medical Illustrators, Guild of Natural Science Illustrators.

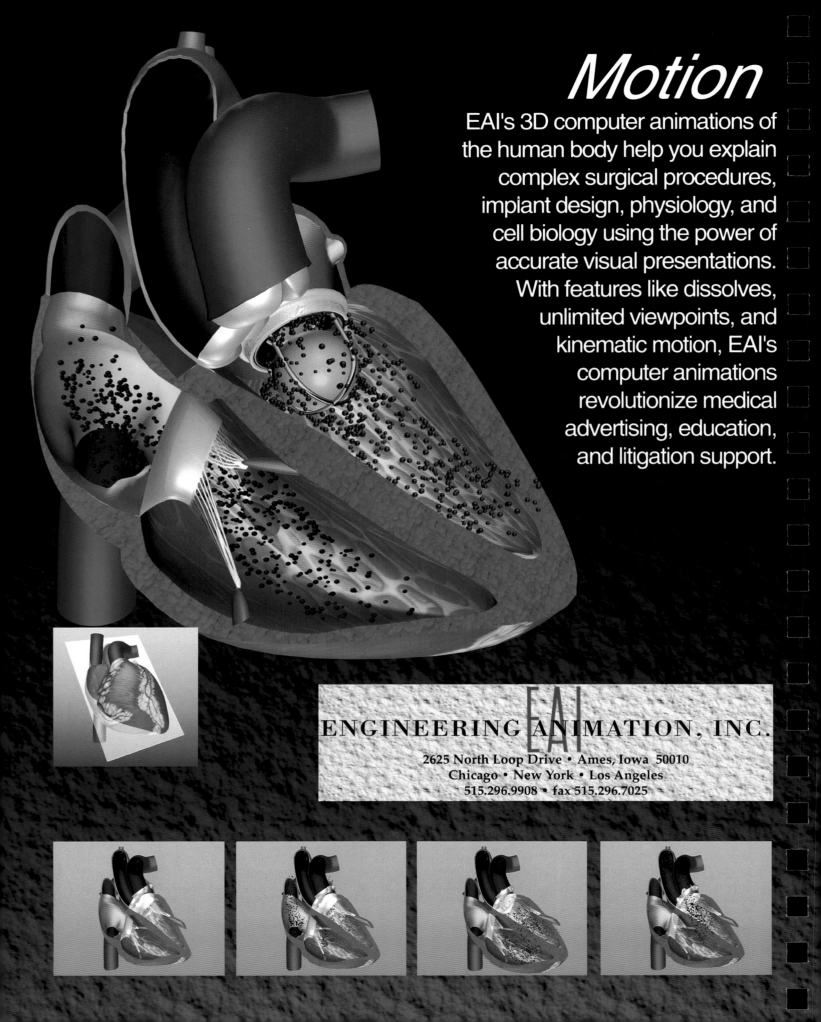

Motion

EAI's 3D computer animations of the human body help you explain complex surgical procedures, implant design, physiology, and cell biology using the power of accurate visual presentations. With features like dissolves, unlimited viewpoints, and kinematic motion, EAI's computer animations revolutionize medical advertising, education, and litigation support.

ENGINEERING **EAI** ANIMATION, INC.

2625 North Loop Drive • Ames, Iowa 50010
Chicago • New York • Los Angeles
515.296.9908 • fax 515.296.7025

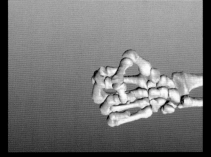

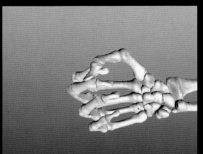

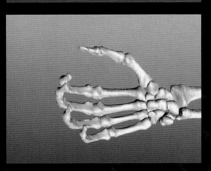

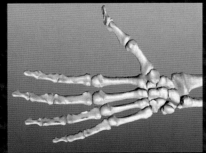

abduct
pronate
constrict
flex
coagulate
rotate
contract
adduct
circulate
supinate
relax

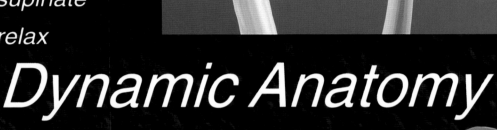

Dynamic Anatomy

ligate
suture
dilate
incise

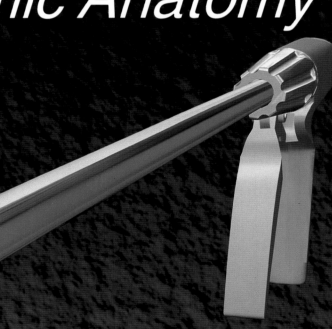

ENGINEERING ANIMATION, INC.
Ames • Chicago • New York • Los Angeles
800.EAI.6777
Call for a Free Demo Tape

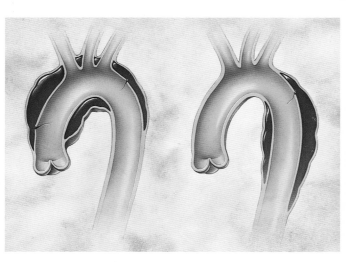

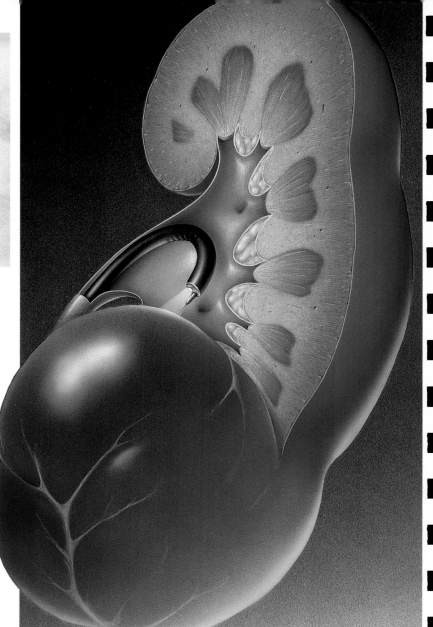

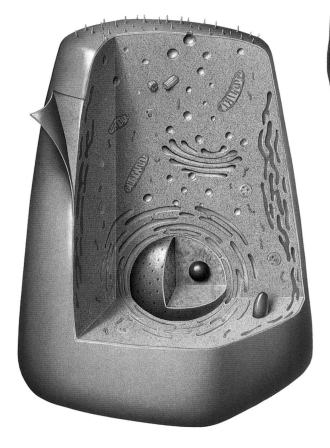

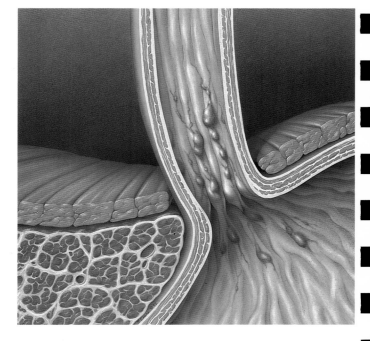

BRIAN EVANS ILLUSTRATION, INC.

1304 PONDEROSA DRIVE FORT COLLINS CO 80521   303.482.7653

BRIAN EVANS MS CMI   MEDICAL ART FOR EDITORIAL USE, TEXTBOOKS, PATIENT EDUCATION, AND ADVERTISING

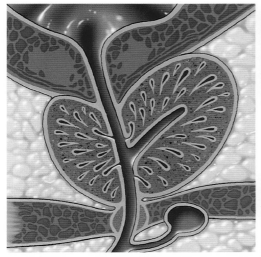
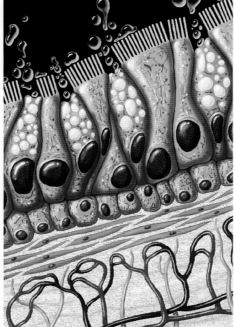
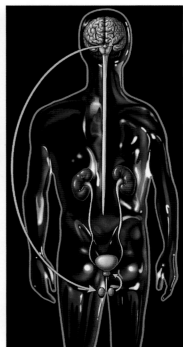
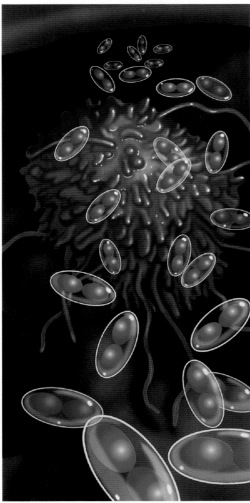
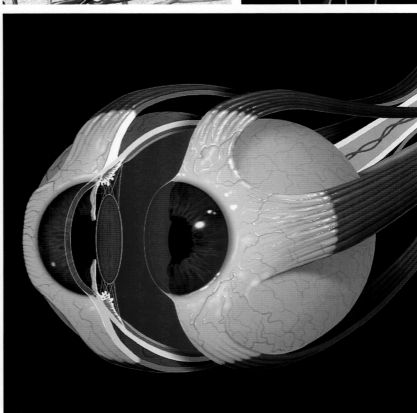

242-09 43rd Avenue
Douglaston, NY 11363
Phone/FAX (718) 279-1659

Medical illustration for print, video or computer-based training programs.

B.A., Fine Art (with Highest Honors), Middlebury College, 1979. M.A. (A.B.T.), Biomedical Communications, The University of Texas Health Science Center at Dallas, 1982. Full-time medical illustrator for pharmaceutical consulting firm 1982–1987. Full-time freelance since 1987. Painting with computers 1991 to present.

Four Association of Medical Illustrators Awards, One HeSCA Award, Exhibitor at Rx Club Shows.

Board Certified Medical Illustrator. Member of the Association of Medical Illustrators since 1982.

AUDRA GERAS

(416) 928-2965, Fax (416) 960-4734

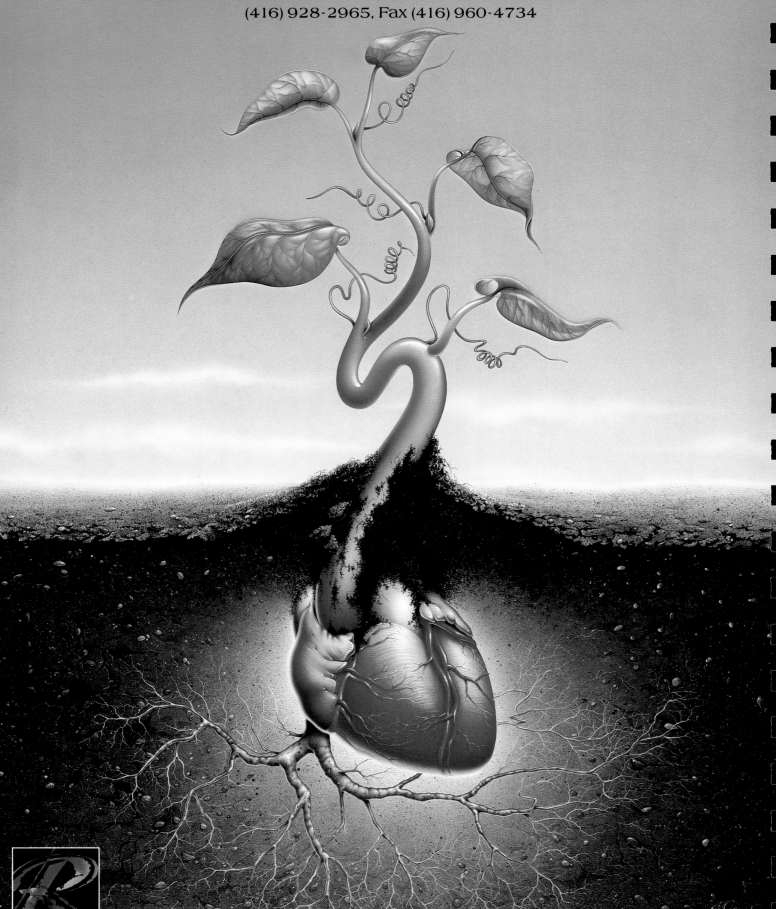

REPRESENTED BY: RENARD REPRESENTS INC. (212) 490-2450 • FAX (212) 697-6828

AUDRA GERAS

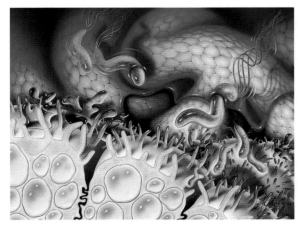

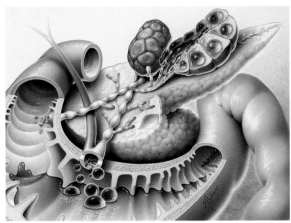

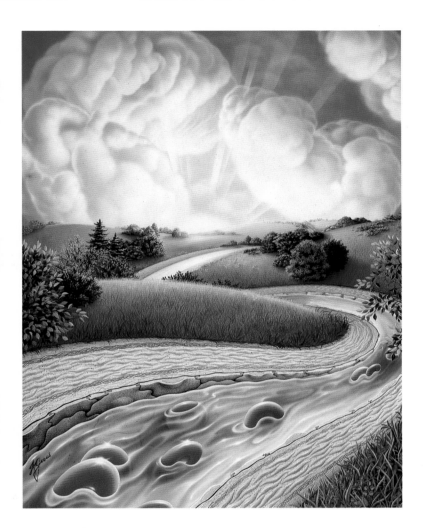

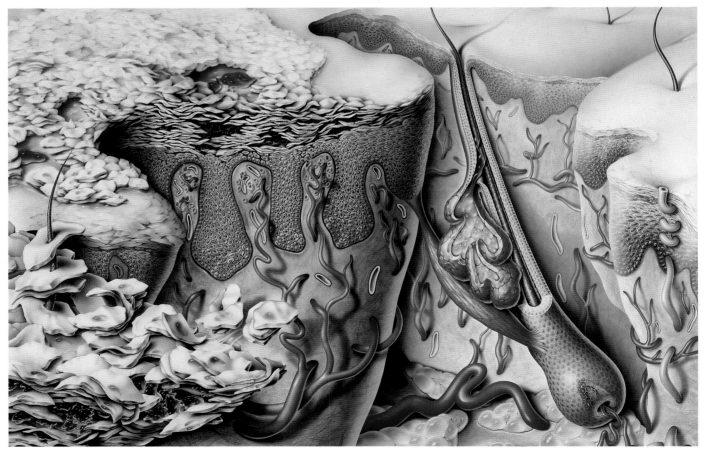

REPRESENTED BY: RENARD REPRESENTS INC. (212) 490-2450 • FAX (212) 697-6828

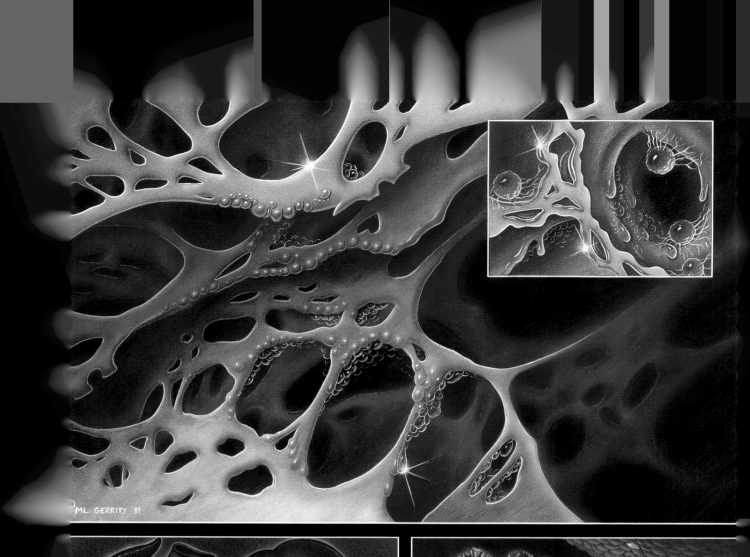

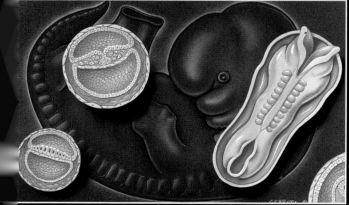

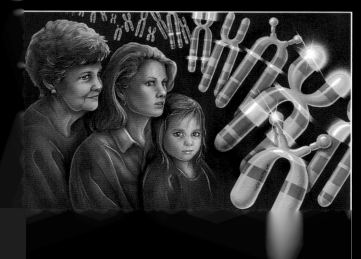

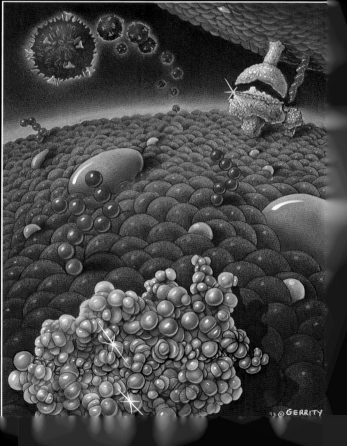

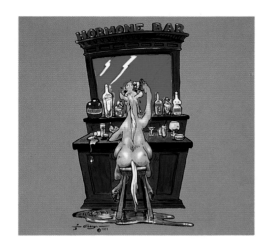

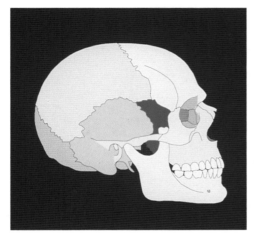

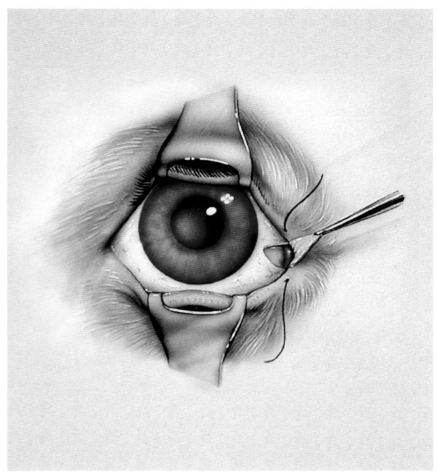

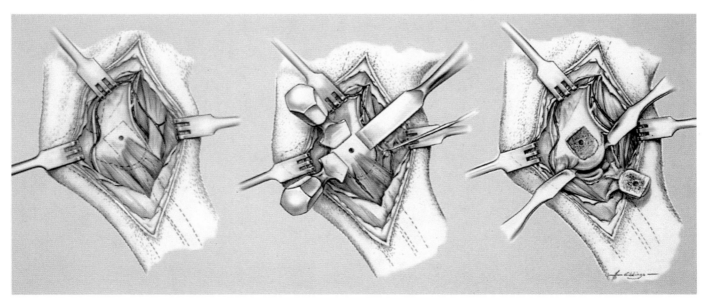

GIDDINGS STUDIO & PUBLICATION

F.D. Giddings
5913 Greenridge Circle
Fort Collins, CO 80525
(303) 226-8587   FAX (303) 491-7907

AREAS OF SPECIALIZATION: Medical:
Human and Veterinary medicine, Ophthalmology (4 texts published); Orthopedics (3 texts
published); Anatomy (4 texts published).
Research: Neurobiology; Electron Microscopy.

CLIENTS: W.B. Saunders Publishing; C.V.
Mosby, Churchill-Livingstone; Colorado State
University, Clinical Science Dept., Anatomy
Dept., Biochemistry Dept., and Biology
Department.

PROFESSIONAL BACKGROUND: Master's
degree (MS) in Anatomy, 1974. AMI Membership, 1974. Illustrating books in biology,
medicine and veterinary medicine since 1960.

PROFESSIONAL MEMBERSHIPS: AMI,
Publisher's Marketing Association, Graphic

Artist's Guild and Society of Children's Book
Writers and Illustrators.

AWARDS/HONORS: 1993 Award of Excel-
lence for "Atlas of Surgical Approaches to the
Bones and Joints of the Dog & Cat," W.B.
Saunders.

OTHER: Established a Medical Illustration
teaching program at Colorado State University
in 1974. Accredited in 1985/86, it was dropped
from the curriculum due to budget cuts.

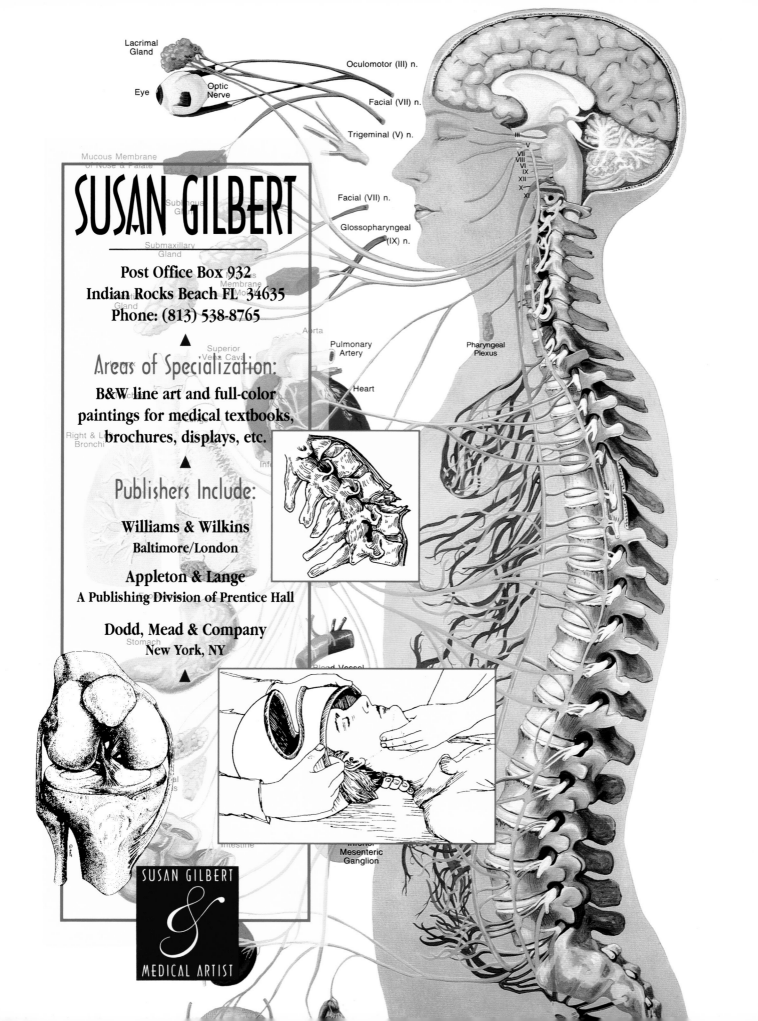

SUSAN GILBERT

Post Office Box 932
Indian Rocks Beach FL 34635
Phone: (813) 538-8765

▲

Areas of Specialization:

B&W line art and full-color paintings for medical textbooks, brochures, displays, etc.

▲

Publishers Include:

Williams & Wilkins
Baltimore/London

Appleton & Lange
A Publishing Division of Prentice Hall

Dodd, Mead & Company
New York, NY

▲

SUSAN GILBERT
&
MEDICAL ARTIST

Anne B. Greene

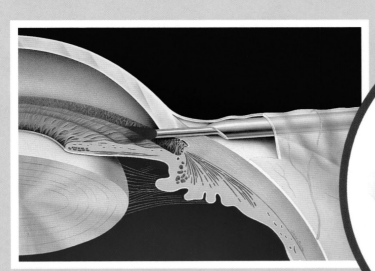

Laser Sclerostomy

Facial Anatomy

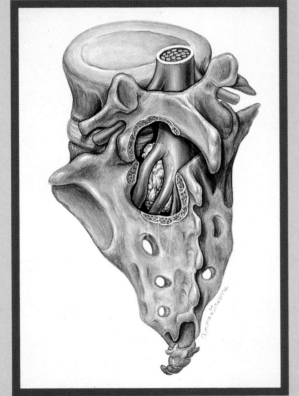

Herniated Disc

COMPLEMENT CASCADE

Anne B. Greene

Certified Medical Illustrator

70 Rocky Pond Road
Boylston, MA 01505
Telephone & Fax:
(508) 869-6440

- More than 20 years' experience as a freelancer; former staff illustrator for the Lahey Clinic

- Ability to communicate clearly as a result of extensive background in biological research

HAKOLA STUDIO

SUSAN HAKOLA

Medical and Scientific Illustration
16990 Martin-Welch Road
Marysville, Ohio 43040
(513)642-2837

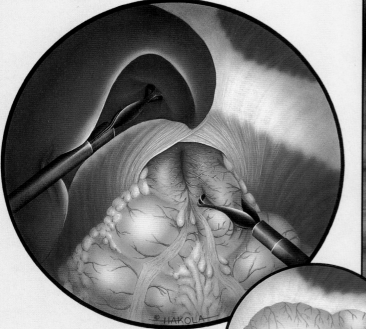

Laparoscopic hiatal
hernia repair

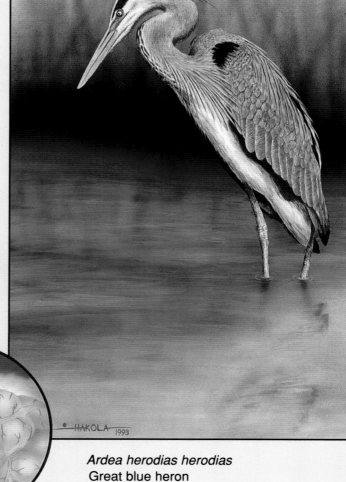

Ardea herodias herodias
Great blue heron

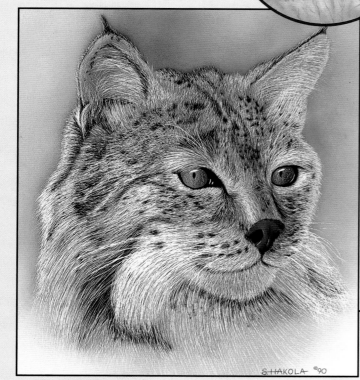

Lynx rufus, California Bobcat

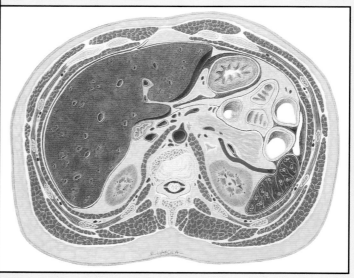

Abdominal cross-section at the level
of T-12, viewed caudal to cephalad

Curriculum vitae and portfolio samples
are available on request.

ENID
HATTON

TEL. (203) 259-3789 • FAX (203) 254-2019
46 PARKWAY • FAIRFIELD, CT 06430

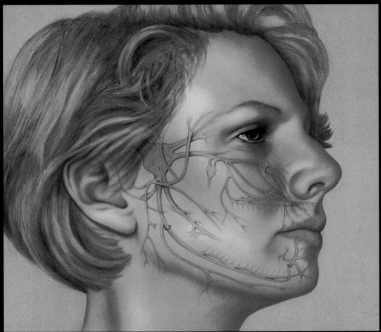

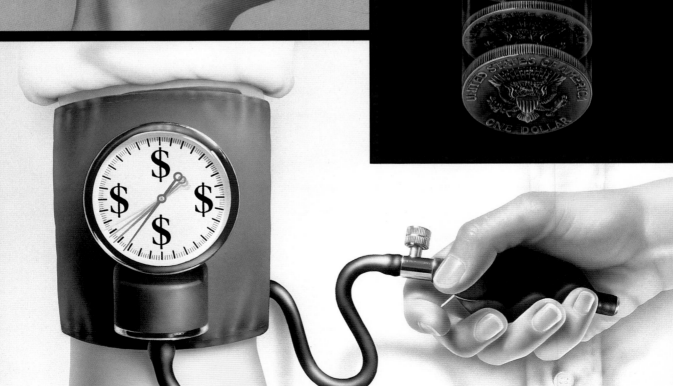

Printed with the permission of Ciba-Geigy Pharmaceutical.

Printed with the permission of Ciba-Geigy Pharmaceutical.

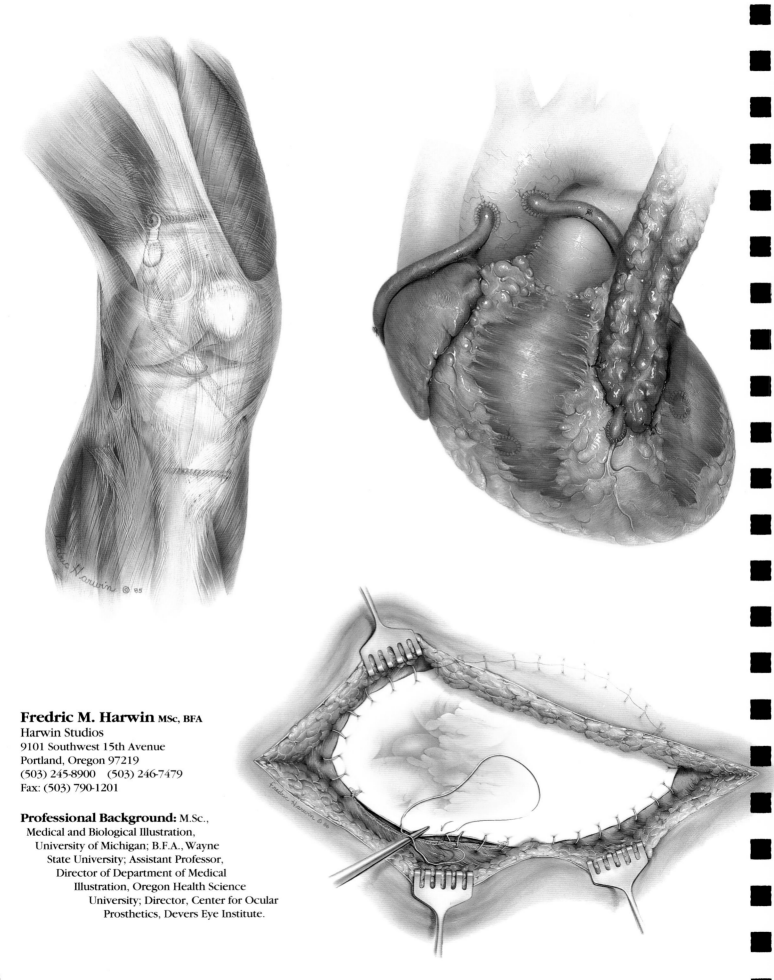

Fredric M. Harwin MSc, BFA
Harwin Studios
9101 Southwest 15th Avenue
Portland, Oregon 97219
(503) 245-8900   (503) 246-7479
Fax: (503) 790-1201

Professional Background: M.Sc.,
  Medical and Biological Illustration,
    University of Michigan; B.F.A., Wayne
      State University; Assistant Professor,
        Director of Department of Medical
          Illustration, Oregon Health Science
            University; Director, Center for Ocular
              Prosthetics, Devers Eye Institute.

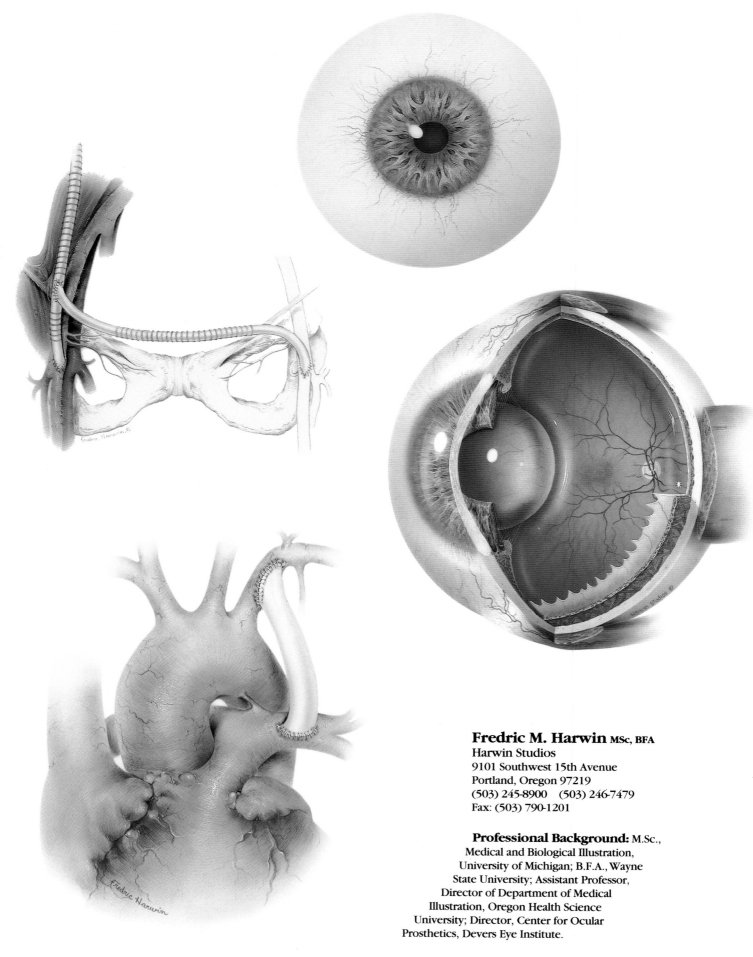

Fredric M. Harwin MSc, BFA
Harwin Studios
9101 Southwest 15th Avenue
Portland, Oregon 97219
(503) 245-8900   (503) 246-7479
Fax: (503) 790-1201

Professional Background: M.Sc.,
Medical and Biological Illustration,
University of Michigan; B.F.A., Wayne
State University; Assistant Professor,
Director of Department of Medical
Illustration, Oregon Health Science
University; Director, Center for Ocular
Prosthetics, Devers Eye Institute.

JACKIE HEDA
MEDICAL ILLUSTRATION

(704) 543-6721 • FAX (704) 543-6873

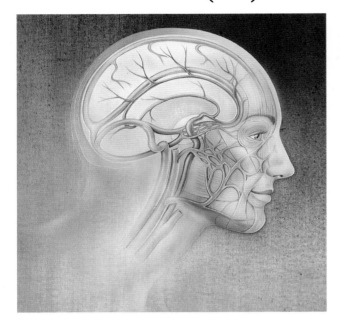

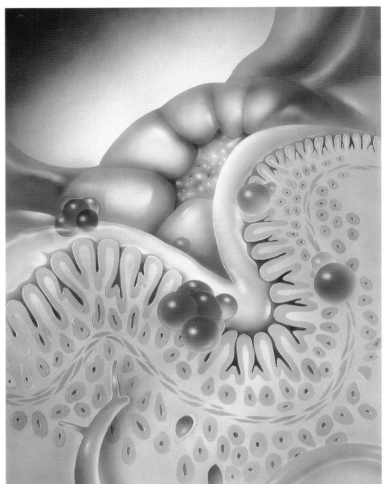

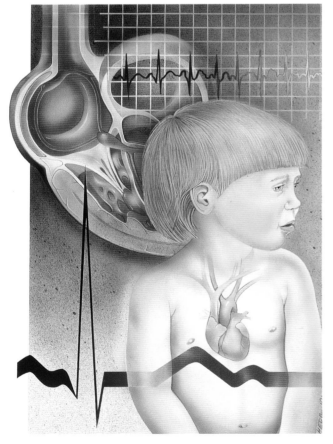

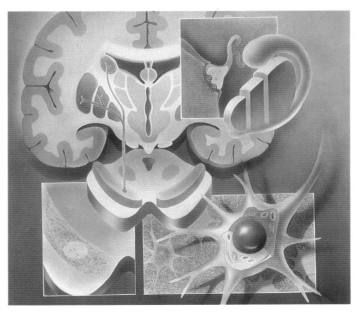

4800 QUAIL CANYON DRIVE • CHARLOTTE, NC 28226

JACKIE HEDA
MEDICAL ILLUSTRATION

(704) 543-6721 • FAX (704) 543-6873

Printed with the permission of Wedgewood Communications

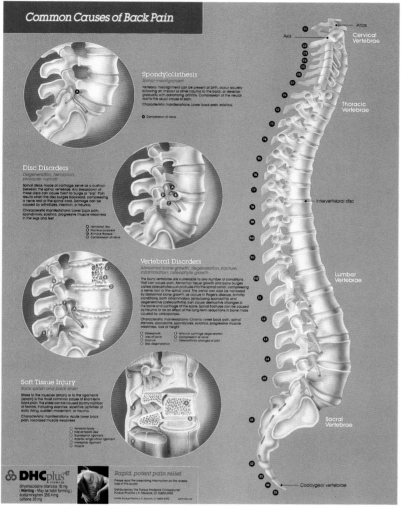

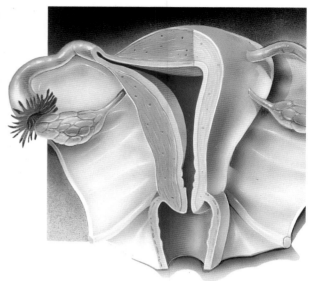

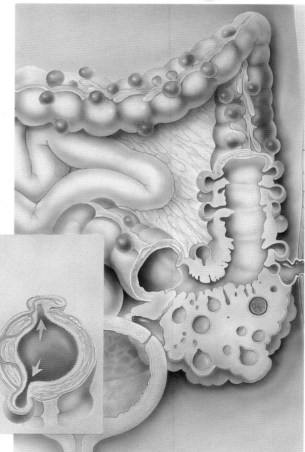

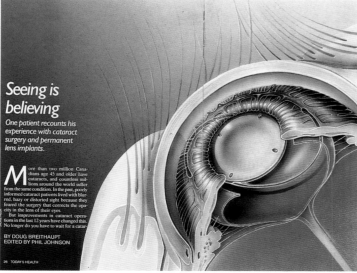

4800 QUAIL CANYON DRIVE • CHARLOTTE, NC 28226

JONATHAN HERBERT

STATE-OF-THE-ART
3D MODELING
FOR PRINT AND
ANIMATION.
CALL FOR BOOK
OR REEL

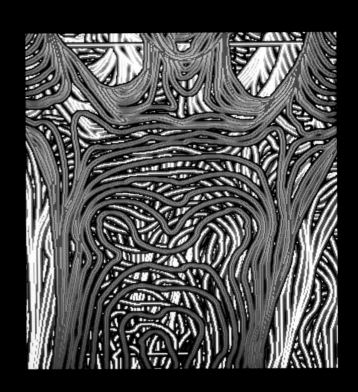

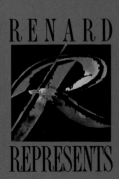

RENARD
REPRESENTS

TEL: 212•490•2450
FAX: 212•697•6828

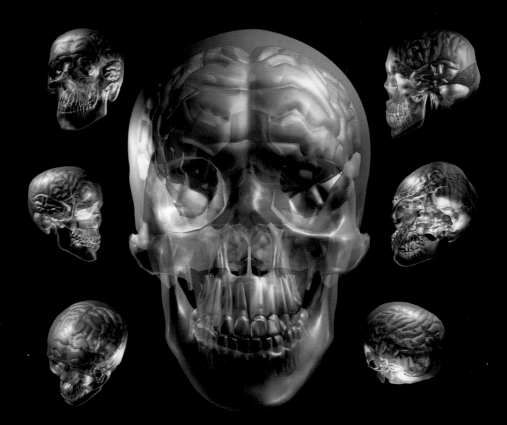

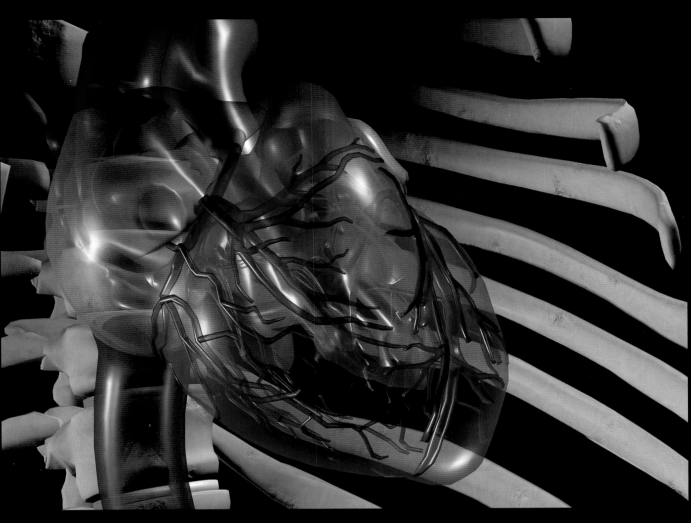

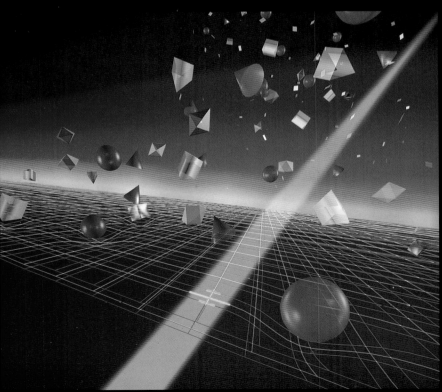

© 1994 Jonathan Herbert

COMPUTER Illustration

TEL: 212•490•2450
FAX: 212•697•6828

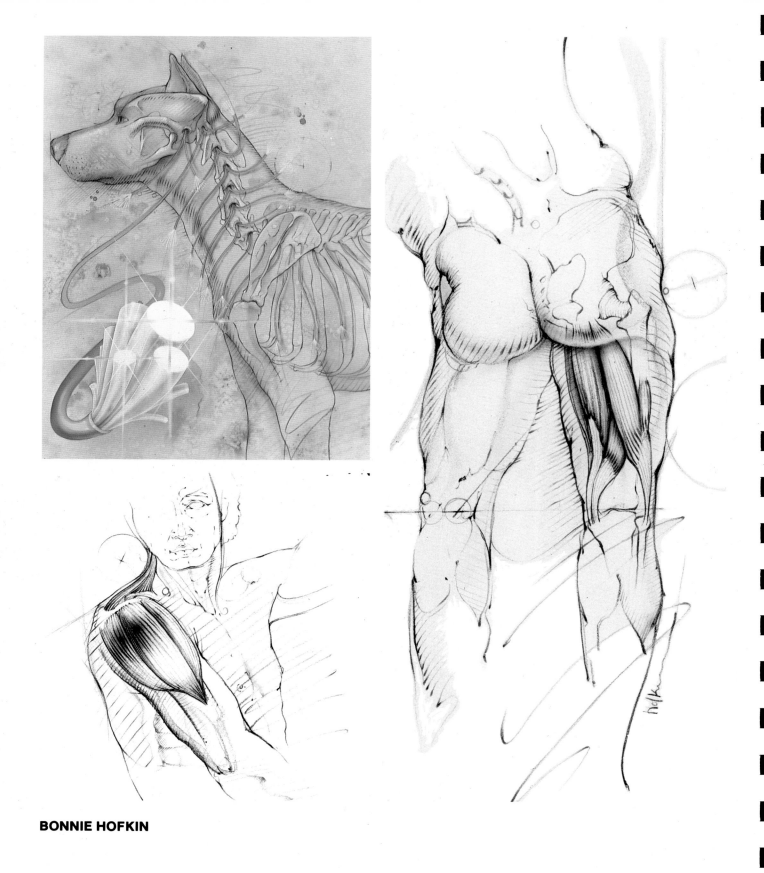

BONNIE HOFKIN

Represented by Joanne Palulian
18 McKinley Street
Rowayton, Connecticut 06853
(212) 581-8338
(203) 866-3734
FAX (203) 857-0842

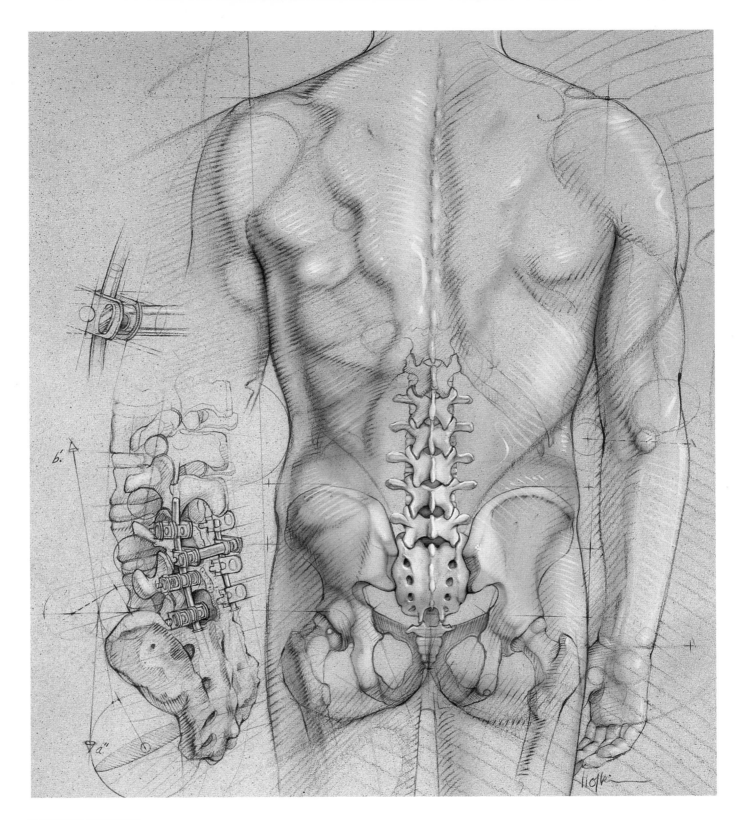

BONNIE HOFKIN

Represented by Joanne Palulian
18 McKinley Street
Rowayton, Connecticut 06853
(212) 581-8338
(203) 866-3734
FAX (203) 857-0842

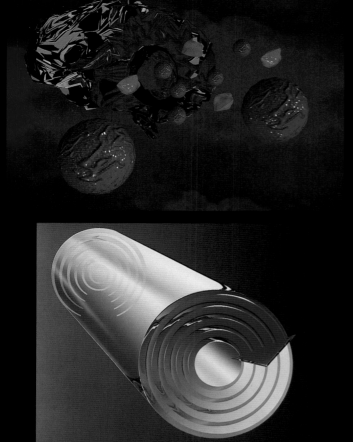

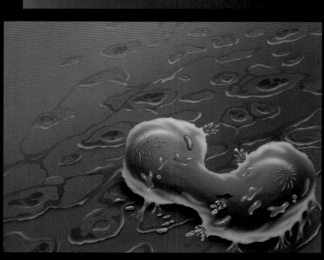

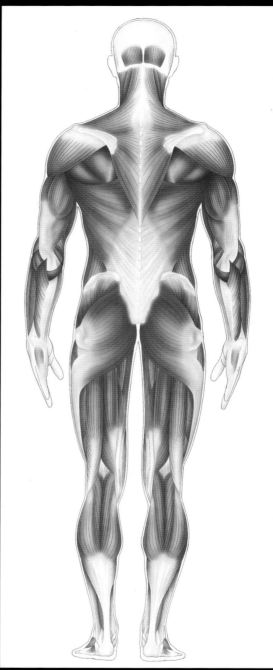

JEFF HOLEWSKI
Jeff Holewski Medico Graphics Inc.
11 Groendyke Circle
Robbinsville, NJ 08691
(609) 443-1497
Beeper (907) 384-2819

AREAS OF SPECIALIZATION: Medical and technical illustration in both airbrush media and computer generated 3-D graphics from presentation comps to final art. Existing art or art to be created can be scanned and manipulated.

CLIENTS: William Douglas McAdams, VICOM/ FCB, Klemtner Advertising, KPR, Medicus Intercon, Harrison Star Wiener & Beitler, Blunt Hann Sersen, and Thomas Ferguson Associates. Serving such accounts as: Hoffman La Roche, Glaxo,

Searle, Dupont, Pharmacia, and Ortho Pharmaceuticals.

PROFESSIONAL BACKGROUND: Fourteen years freelance experience. President Jeff Holewski Medico Graphics Inc.

PROFESSIONAL MEMBERSHIPS: AMI.

AWARDS/HONORS: Awards of Excellence, Rx Club 1989, 1990, 1991, 1993.

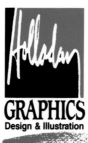

GRAPHICS
Design & Illustration

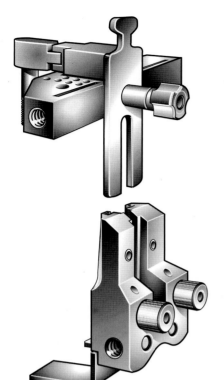

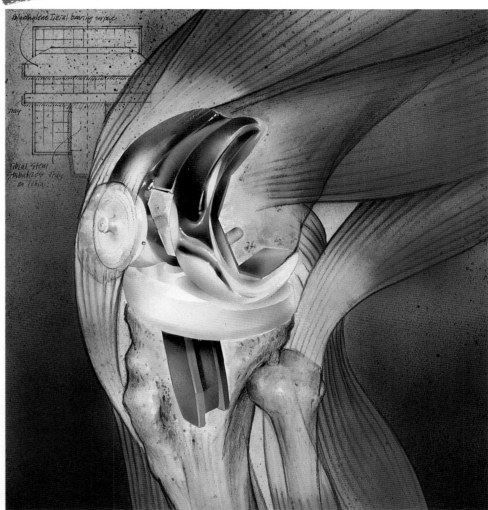

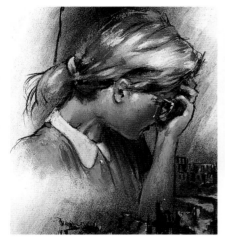

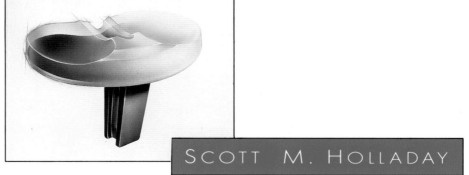

SCOTT M. HOLLADAY

1504 East Main Street • Warsaw, Indiana 46580 • Phone: 219-269-6466 • Fax: 219-269-1665

Floyd E. Hosmer

Certified Medical Illustrator

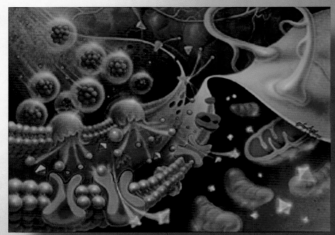

Nerve Synapse

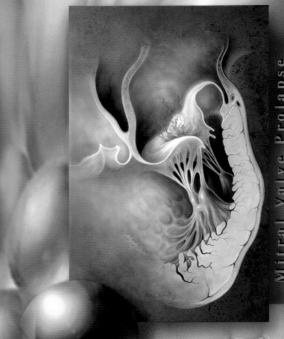

Mitral Valve Prolapse

1860 Cedarwood Road
Birmingham, Alabama 35216
TEL (205) 979-8317
FAX (205) 979-3275

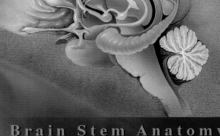

Brain Stem Anatomy

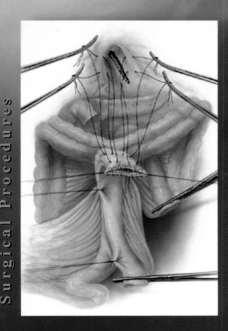

Surgical Procedures

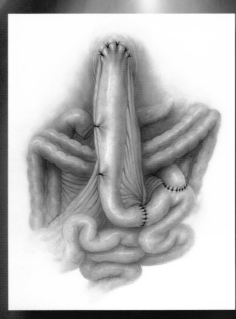

- Conceptuals
- Surgery
- Patient Education
- Biological
- Pharmaceutical
- Anatomical
- Editorial
- Line
- Continuous Tone
- Color

Floyd E. Hosmer

Certified Medical Illustrator

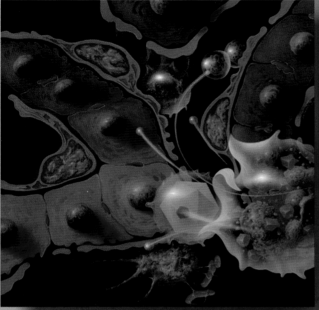

Infection Within Liver Cells

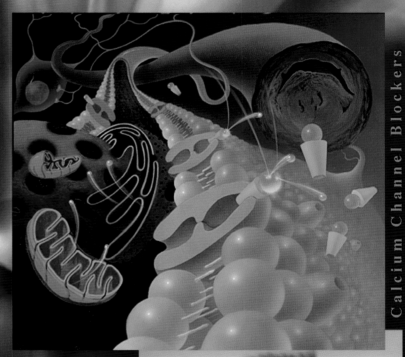

Calcium Channel Blockers

1860 Cedarwood road
Birmingham, Alabama 35216

TEL (205) 979-8317
FAX (205) 979-3275

Editorial

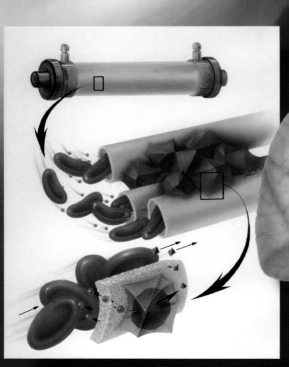

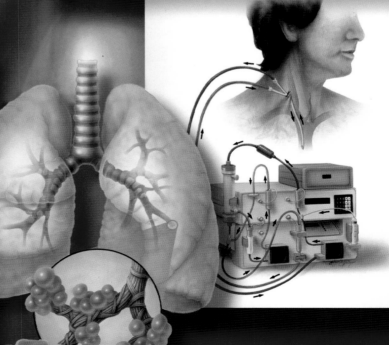

Anatomy of the
Alveoli in the Lungs

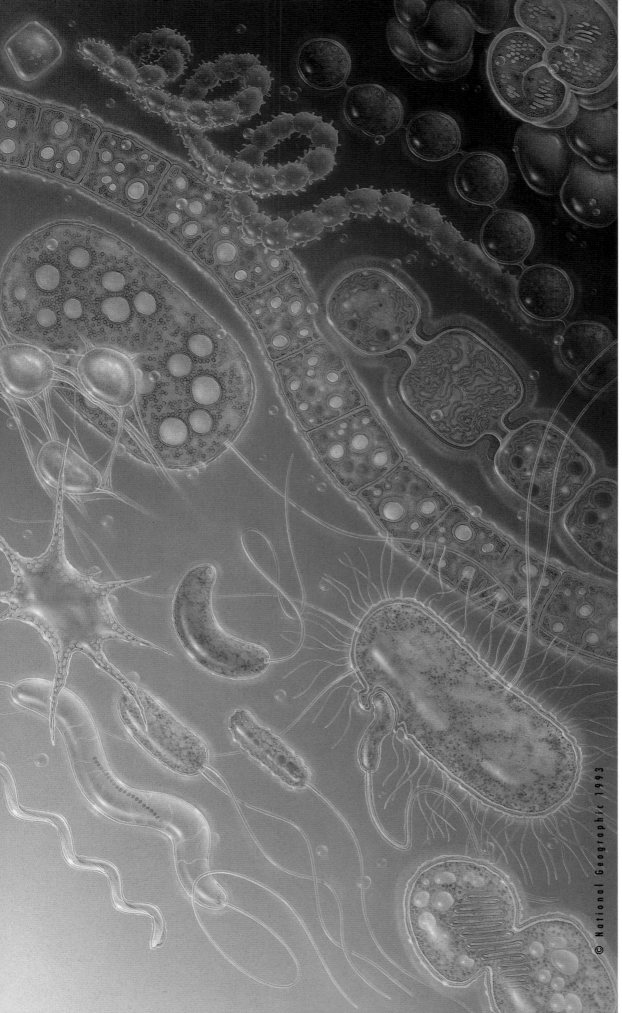

JANE HURD

351 Pacific Street
Brooklyn, NY 11217

Tel: (718) 624-7174
Tel: (212) 556-5167
Fax: (212) 556-5181

*Over 20 years
experience in
medical illustration.
BS with honors in
medical art from
Univ of Illinois.
Twenty-two awards
from AMI.*

Stock art also
available:

Normal Heart

Coronary Bypass

Hypercholesterolemia

Pediatric Heart Exam

Childhood UTI

Normal Lungs

COPD

Allergy/H2Blockers

CO Poisoning

Headache

Spina Bifida

Osteoporosis

Office GYN

Endometrial Cancer

Stages of Labor

Gastric Ulcer

Knee Joint

Arthritis

Office Lab

Genetics

Gene Gate

© National Geographic 1993

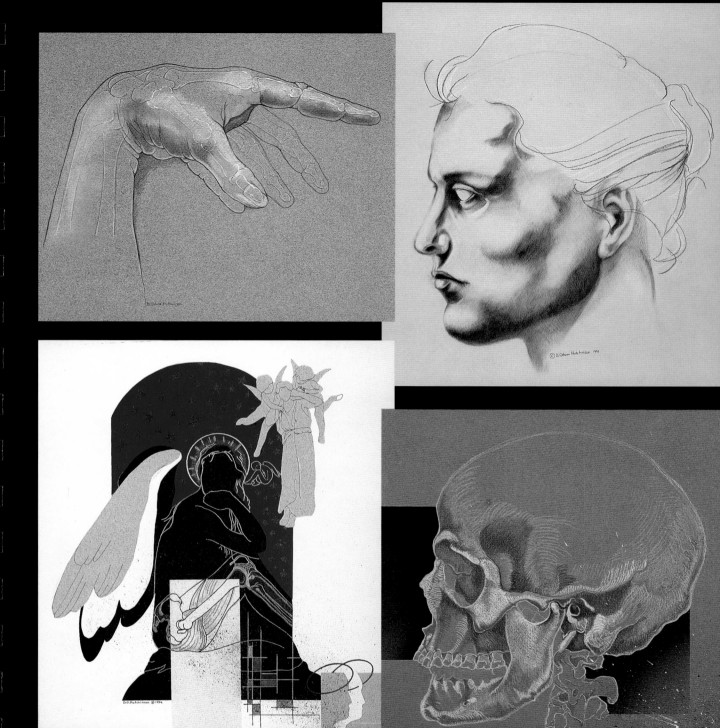

DEBORAH ODUM HUTCHINSON
Southern Rim Graphics
9046 Oak Hill Circle
College Station, TX 77845
(409) 846-1230

AREAS OF SPECIALIZATION: Black and
white and full-color conceptual illustration for
medical, editorial, advertising and fine arts.
Watercolor, colored pencils, pastels, pen and
ink and airbrush.

CLIENTS: Publishers of medical and scientific
textbooks and periodicals, pharmaceutical
advertising agencies: B.C. Decker Pub., Co.;
Upjohn Pharmaceutical Corp.; Waltman and
Associates; Memorial Hospital System; Fahlgren
Martin advertising; RCW Communication
Design, Inc.; Medical Economics Pub., Co.

PROFESSIONAL BACKGROUND: Over 12
years experience as a medical illustrator for
Texas A&M University, College of Medicine.
Currently a full-time freelance artist.

PROFESSIONAL MEMBERSHIPS: Association of Medical Illustrators.

AWARDS/HONORS: AMI Certificate of Merit,
1991; Solo exhibitions 1991–1993, The College
of Medicine, Texas A&M University; Mostra di
Pittura, Santa Chiara, Castiglion Fiorentino, Italy.

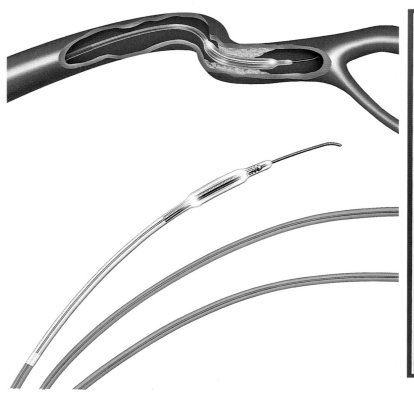

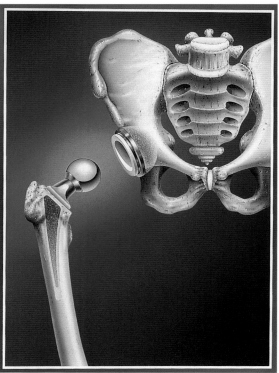

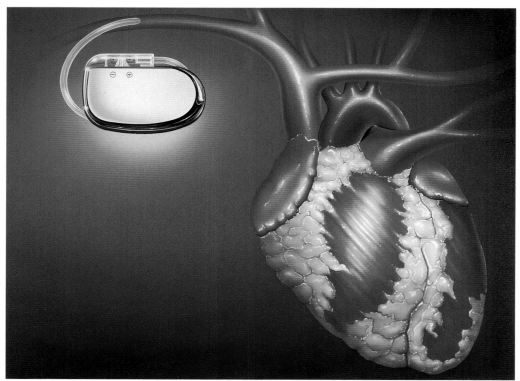

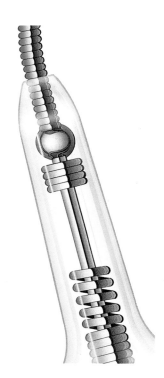

J o h n H u x t a b l e
I l l u s t r a t i o n

Areas Of Specialization:
Anatomical, surgical, biological,
and product illustration with
emphasis on highly detailed and
technical illustrations.

Kathy Braun Represents
1-800-755-3380

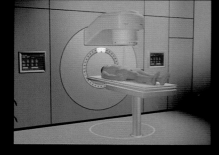
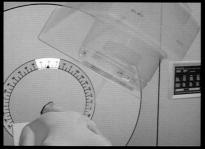
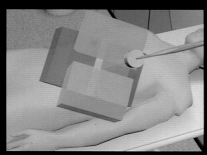
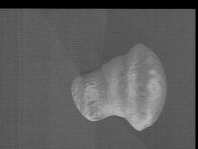
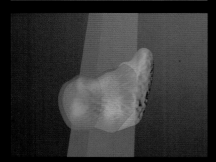

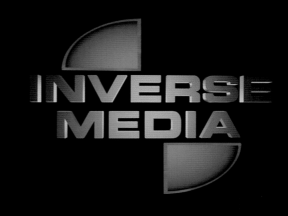

INVERSE MEDIA

COMPUTER ANIMATION

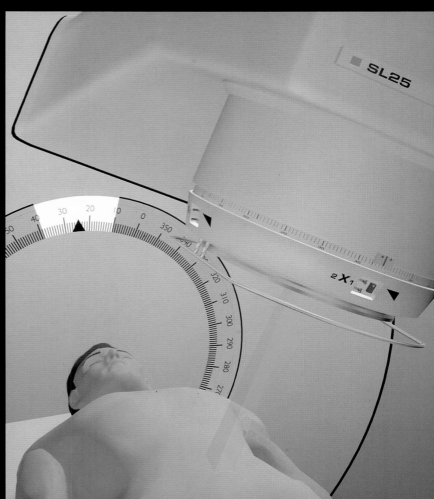

INVERSE MEDIA
Christopher Thomas
500 Pequot Court
PO Box 1072
Southport, CT 06490
(203) 255-9620
FAX (203) 255-9619

COMPUTER ANIMATION:
Inverse Media has specialized in high resolution three-dimensional computer animation for medical and scientific visualization since 1986.

A video demo tape is available upon request.

CLIENTS:
Burroughs Wellcome, Boehringer Ingelheim, Davis & Geck, Philips Medical, Schering.

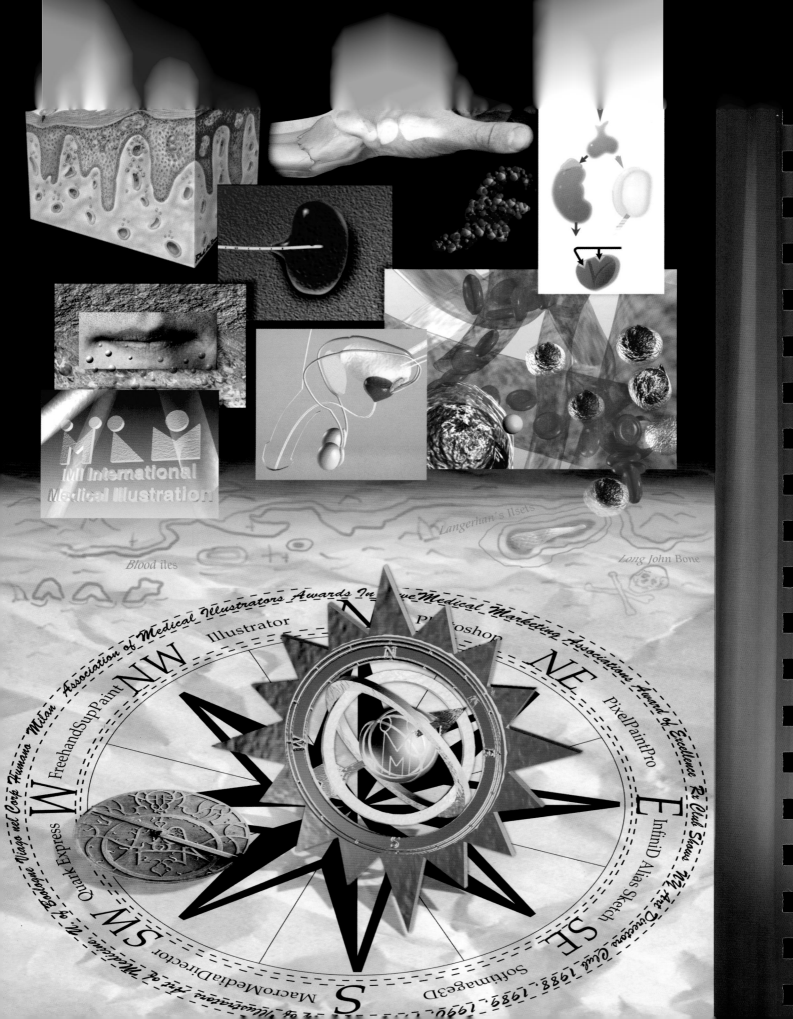

IMI Illustrations 1-800 665-0781

In Canada 514 483-5489

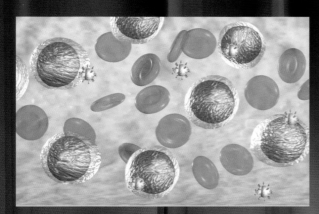

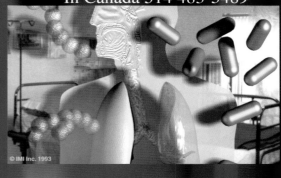

© IMI Inc. 1993

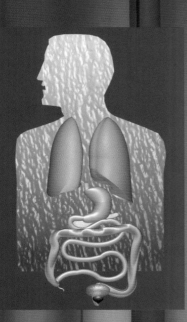

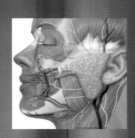

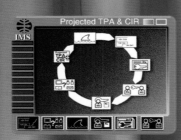

Projected TPA & CIR

IMS

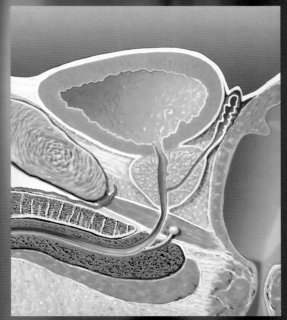

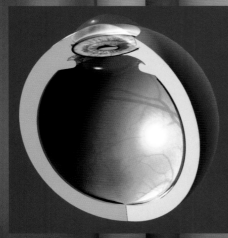

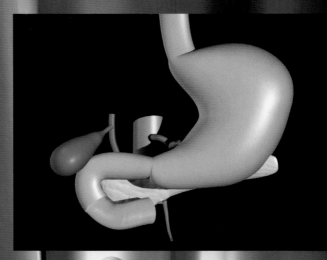

Computer and Traditional
Medical Illustrations for
Publication, Video
and MultiMedia

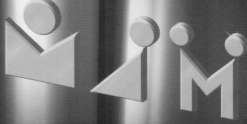

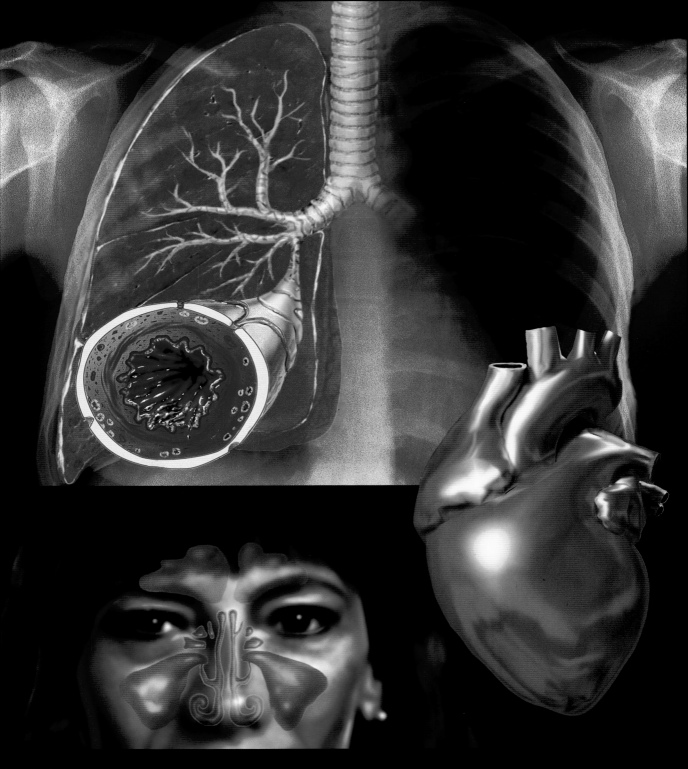

EDWARD M. JONES, C.M.I.
46 Kingsland Circle
Monmouth Junction, NJ 08852
Phone/Fax: (908) 438-0831

AREAS OF SPECIALIZATION: 2D and 3D computer illustration from scratch or in conjunction with scanned images. Can make illustrations look very painterly, photographic or like one-color drawings.

CLIENTS: Ciba, Bristol-Myers Squibb, and through agencies: Lederle, Pfizer Roerig, Eli Lilly, McNeil Pharmaceuticals; others: Merrill Lynch, Medical Economics and companies producing medical products.

PROFESSIONAL BACKGROUND: B.F.A. and M.S. in Medical Illustration from the University of Michigan 1975.

PROFESSIONAL MEMBERSHIPS: A.M.I. and Life Member of the Art Students League in N.Y.C.

SHOWS/AWARDS: Brooklyn Museum, Grand Central Galleries N.Y.C., Levaton Gallery N.Y.C., AMI Awards, Knickerbocker Artist Award N.Y.C.

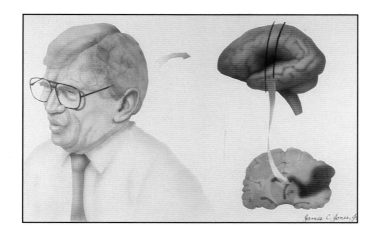

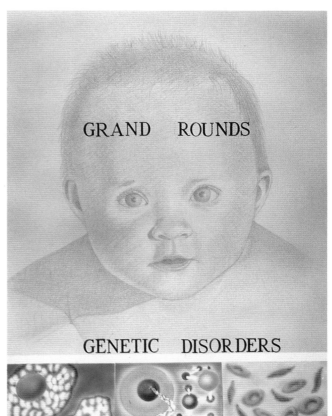

GRAND ROUNDS

GENETIC DISORDERS

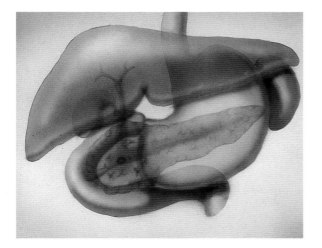

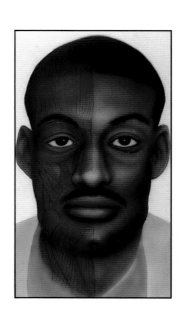

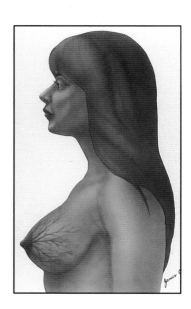

JAMES C. JONES, JR., M.D.

6310 Capon Street
Seat Pleasant, Md. 20743
(301) 350-2487

PROFESSIONAL BACKGROUND:

1983-1987 Graduated from medical school.
Howard University Hospital, Washington, DC.

1987-1988 Awarded a scholarship to the
New York Academy of Art, New York, NY.

1988-1992 Residency in Anatomic and Clinical
Pathology, Howard University Hospital,
Washington, DC.

1992-1993 Fellowship in Clinical Hematology,
Howard University Hospital, Washington, DC.

1993-1994 Fellowship in Transfusion Medicine,
the National Institutes of Health, Bethesda, MD.

PROFESSIONAL MEMBERSHIPS:

American Society of Clinical Pathologists
College of American Pathologists
American Medical Association
Association of American Blood Banks
Association of Medical Illustrators
Association Internationale du Film
Animation (ASIFA-East)

AREAS OF SPECIALIZATION:

Black and white illustrations
Full color airbrushed illustrations
Computer-generated animation

JONES

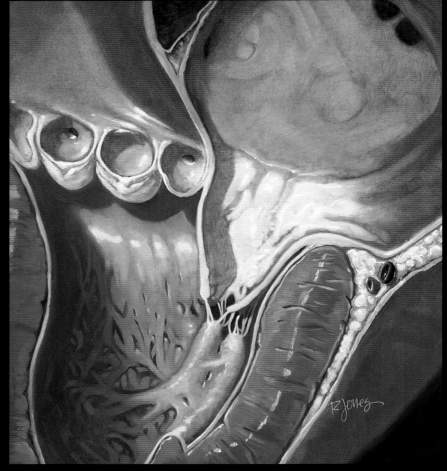

RUSTY JONES
Park Creek Place
3625 N. Hall, Suite 1070
Dallas, Texas 75219
Fax (214) 522-4133
(214) 522-4132

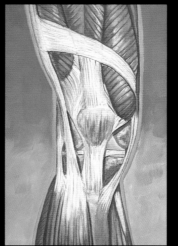

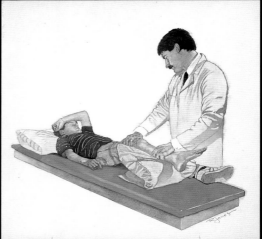

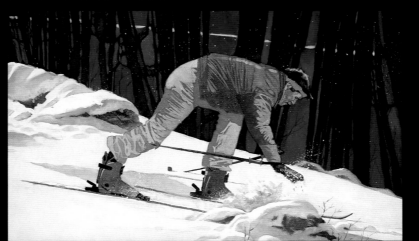

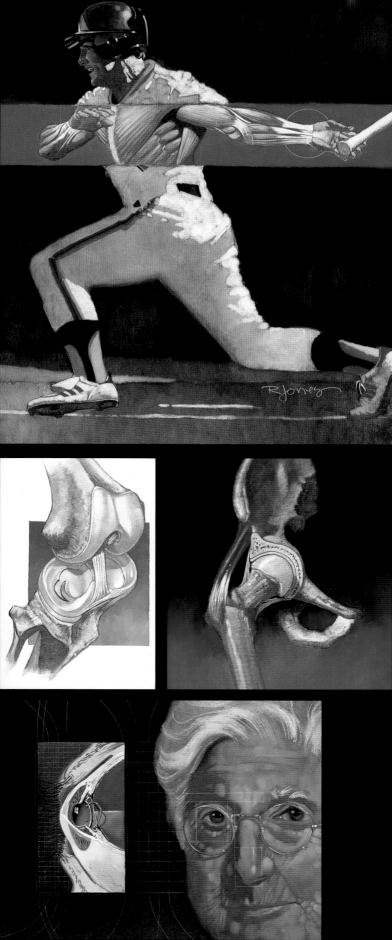

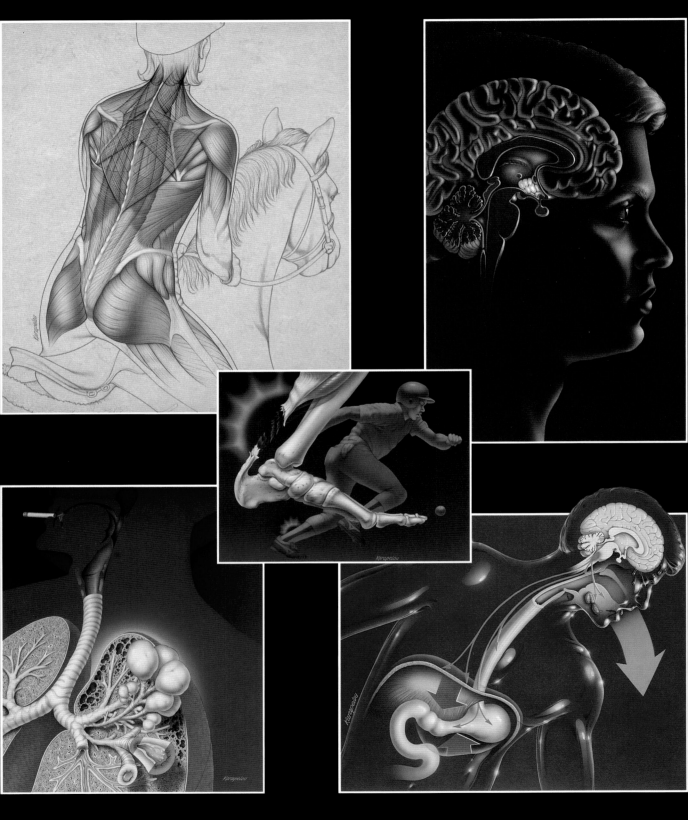

KARAPELOU

John W. Karapelou, CMI

BioMedical Illustrations
3932 Blueberry Hollow Road
Columbus, Ohio 43230
TEL (614) 898-7228 • FAX (614) 898-7322

Creative solutions to visuals communicating science and medicine for advertising, marketing, and publishing.

Over 19 years professional experience. Board certified. B.S. in Medical Illustration. Full-time free-lance practice and Adjunct Instructor, The Ohio State University.

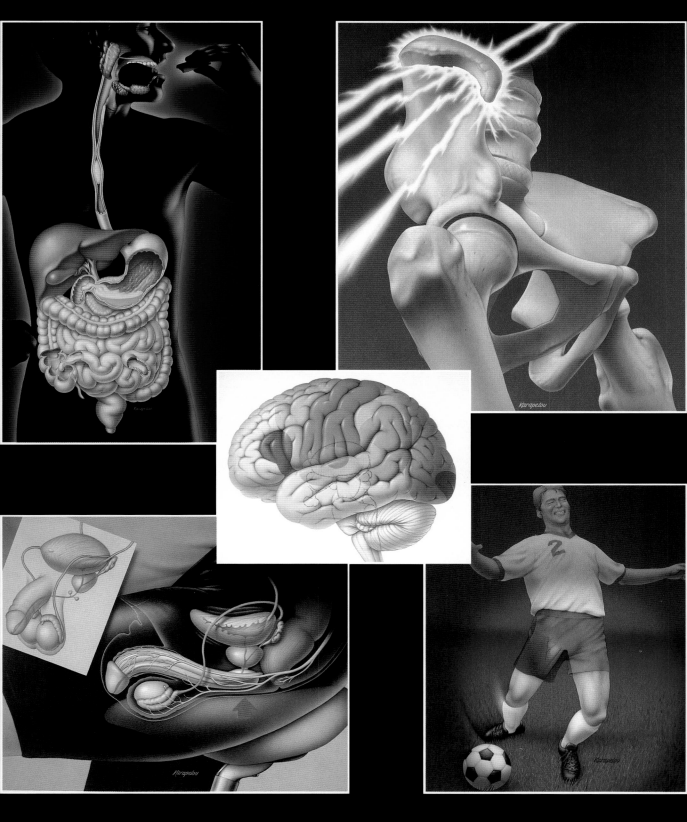

KARAPELOU

Creative solutions to visuals communicating science and medicine for advertising, marketing, and publishing.

A commanding knowledge of human biology enables his award-winning style to maintain the crucial balance between precise scientific accuracy and dramatic impact.

John W. Karapelou, CMI
BioMedical Illustrations
3932 Blueberry Hollow Road
Columbus, Ohio 43230
TEL (614) 898-7228 • FAX (614) 898-7322

KEITH KASNOT

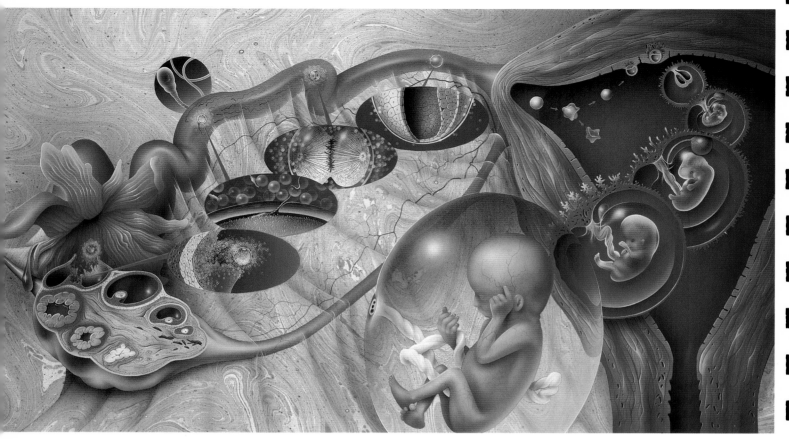

9228 NORTH 29TH STREET

PHOENIX, ARIZONA 85028

TELEPHONE 602.482.6501

FACSIMILE   602.482.6501

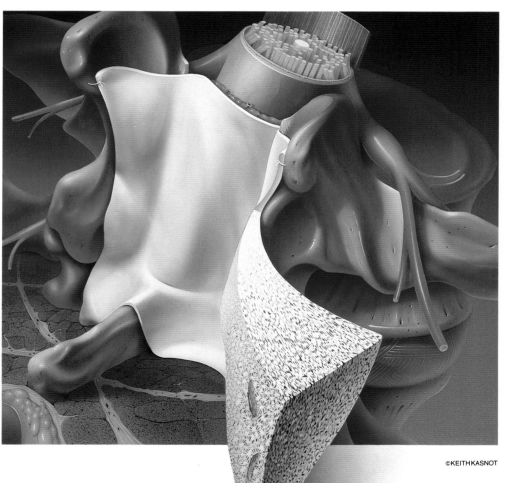

©KEITH KASNOT

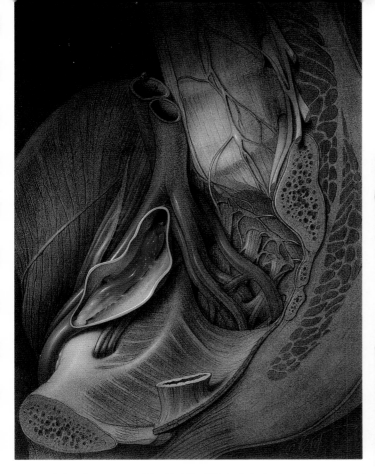

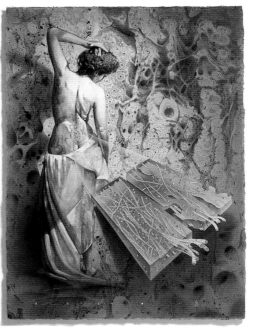

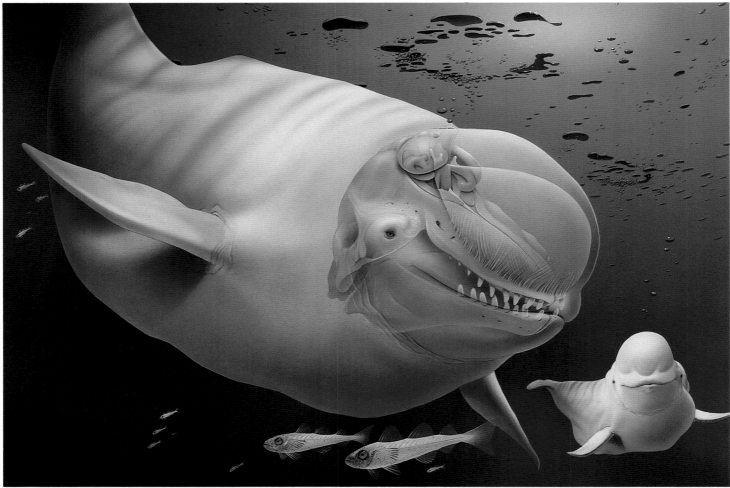

©KEITH KASNOT

121

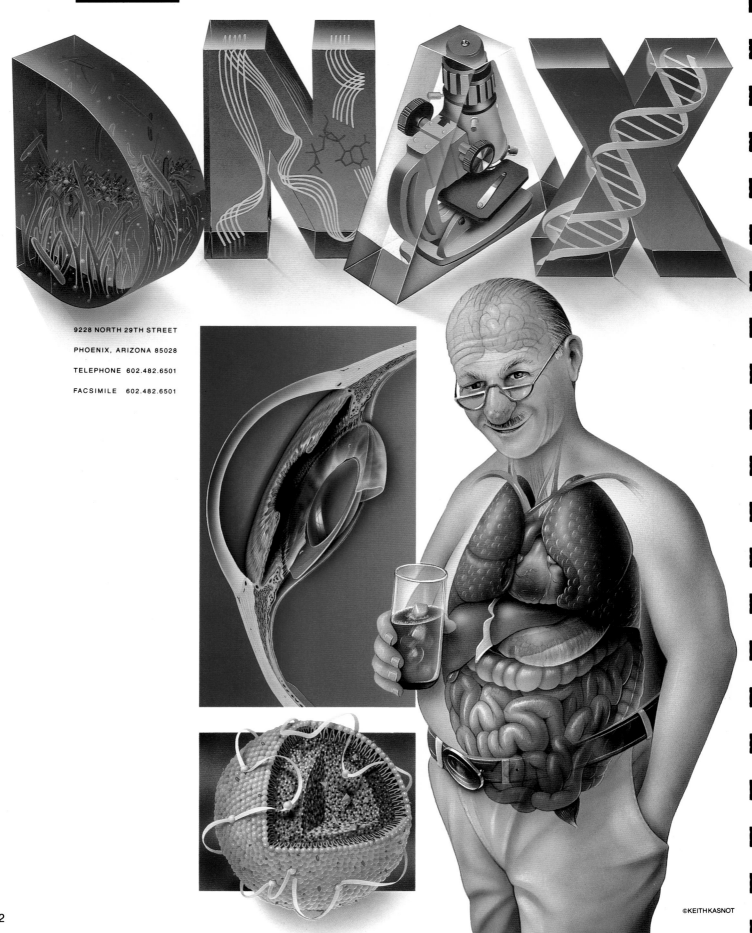

KEITH
KASNOT

9228 NORTH 29TH STREET

PHOENIX, ARIZONA 85028

TELEPHONE 602.482.6501

FACSIMILE 602.482.6501

©KEITHKASNOT

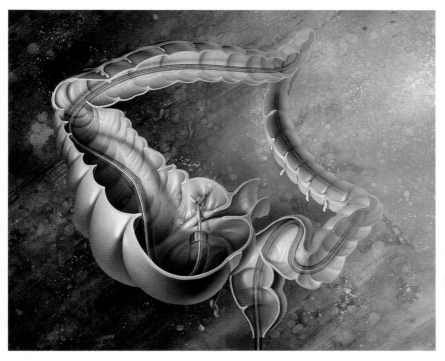

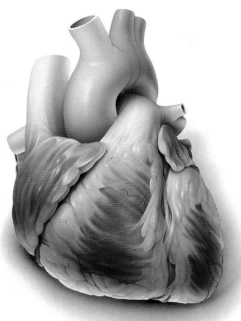

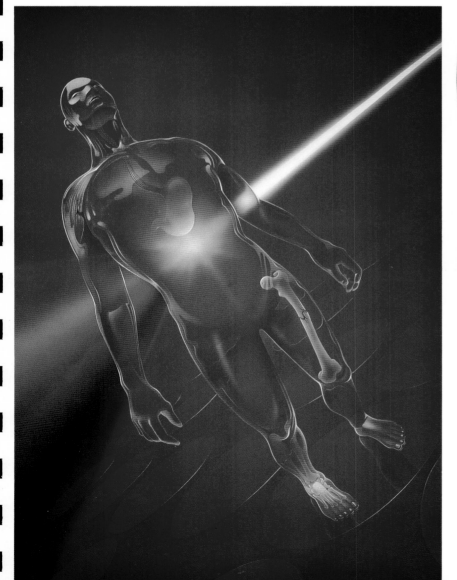

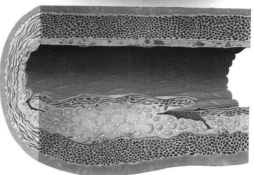

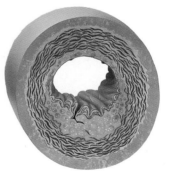

©KEITH KASNOT

CHRISTY KRAMES

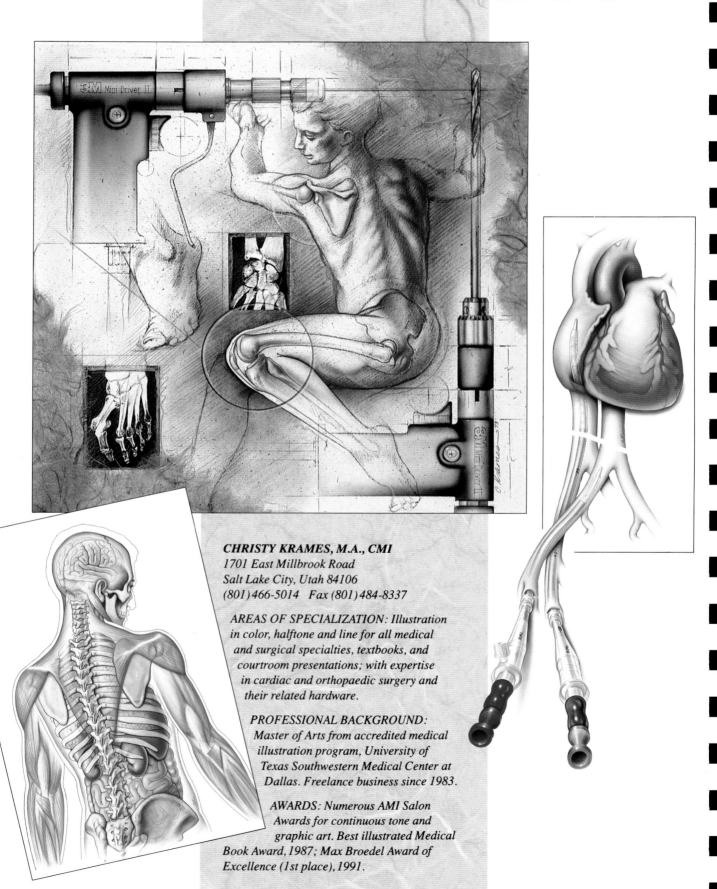

CHRISTY KRAMES, M.A., CMI
1701 East Millbrook Road
Salt Lake City, Utah 84106
(801) 466-5014   Fax (801) 484-8337

*AREAS OF SPECIALIZATION: Illustration
in color, halftone and line for all medical
and surgical specialties, textbooks, and
courtroom presentations; with expertise
in cardiac and orthopaedic surgery and
their related hardware.*

*PROFESSIONAL BACKGROUND:
Master of Arts from accredited medical
illustration program, University of
Texas Southwestern Medical Center at
Dallas. Freelance business since 1983.*

*AWARDS: Numerous AMI Salon
Awards for continuous tone and
graphic art. Best illustrated Medical
Book Award, 1987; Max Broedel Award of
Excellence (1st place), 1991.*

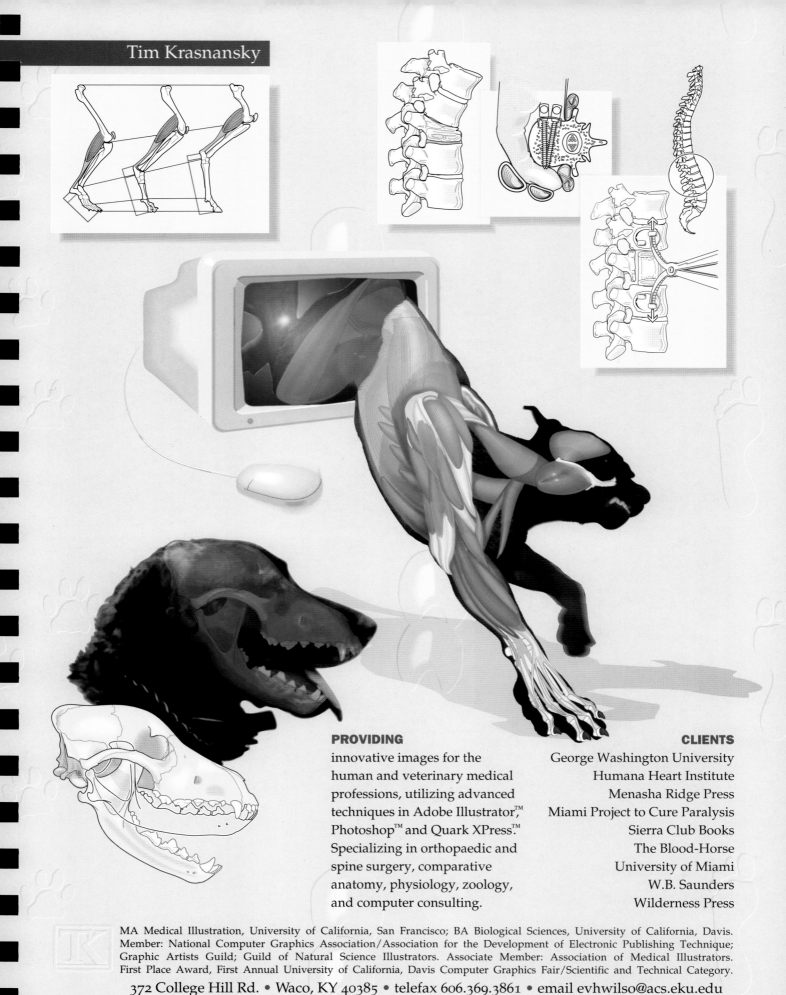

Tim Krasnansky

PROVIDING

innovative images for the human and veterinary medical professions, utilizing advanced techniques in Adobe Illustrator,™ Photoshop™ and Quark XPress™. Specializing in orthopaedic and spine surgery, comparative anatomy, physiology, zoology, and computer consulting.

CLIENTS

George Washington University
Humana Heart Institute
Menasha Ridge Press
Miami Project to Cure Paralysis
Sierra Club Books
The Blood-Horse
University of Miami
W.B. Saunders
Wilderness Press

MA Medical Illustration, University of California, San Francisco; BA Biological Sciences, University of California, Davis. Member: National Computer Graphics Association/Association for the Development of Electronic Publishing Technique; Graphic Artists Guild; Guild of Natural Science Illustrators. Associate Member: Association of Medical Illustrators. First Place Kward, First Annual University of California, Davis Computer Graphics Fair/Scientific and Technical Category.

372 College Hill Rd. • Waco, KY 40385 • telefax 606.369.3861 • email evhwilso@acs.eku.edu

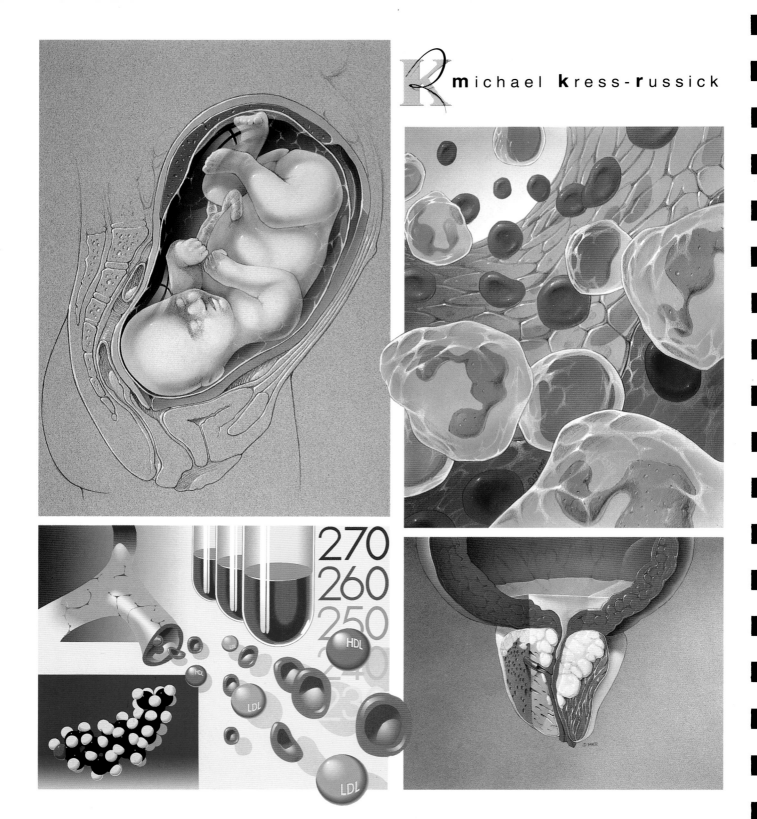

michael kress-russick

MICHAEL KRESS-RUSSICK

2680 A2 Village Green
Aurora, IL 60504
Phone/FAX (708) 820 6211

PROFESSIONAL BACKGROUND: MAMS,
University of Illinois at Chicago.

AREAS OF SPECIALIZATION: Medical art in
line, tone, full color and computer for publication and advertising.

AWARDS/HONORS: AMI Awards of Excellence: 1992 Student Medical Line; 1993
Textbook.

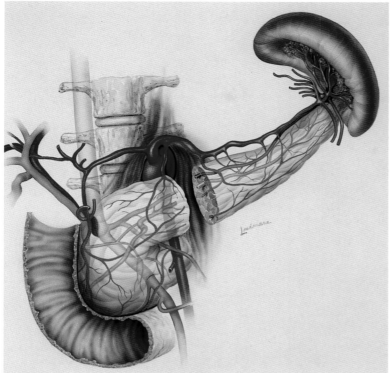

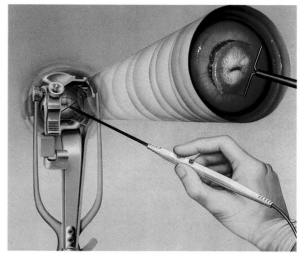

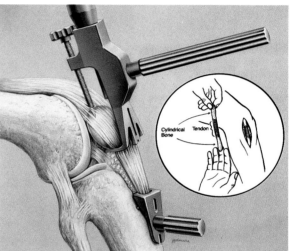

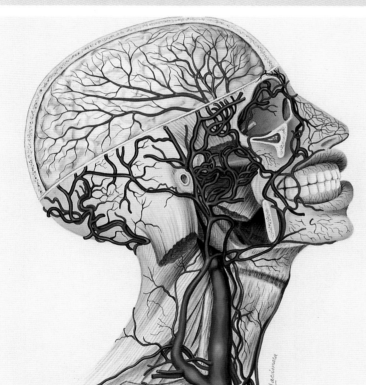

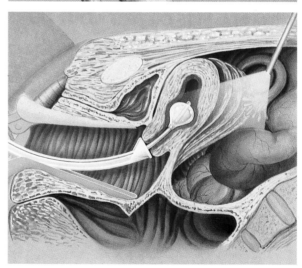

CARLOS LACAMARA STUDIO

22834 Burbank Blvd.
Woodland Hills, CA 91367
(818) 887-5211
FAX (818) 992-7425

AREAS OF SPECIALIZATION: Creating conceptual medical artwork, plus full service art studio for the preparation of ads, logos, brochures, and promotional materials.

CLIENTS: ZINNANTI Surgical Instruments, BEI Medical Systems, TMI TAPCO Medical, Inc., W.J. Medical.

PROFESSIONAL BACKGROUND: Over 30 years of experience creating artwork for the medical industry as well as for nature, aerospace and historic projects. Several years with *National Geographic* magazine.

PROFESSIONAL MEMBERSHIPS: Association of Medical Illustrators.

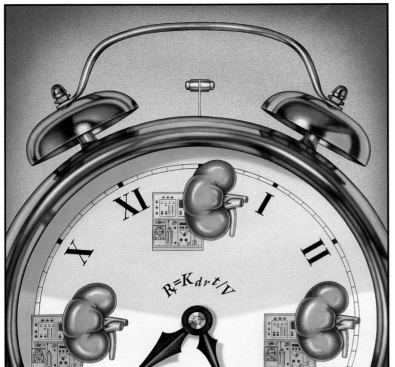

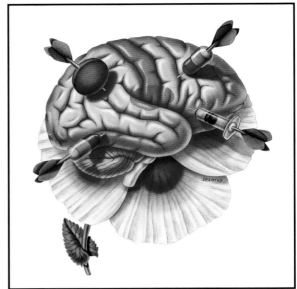

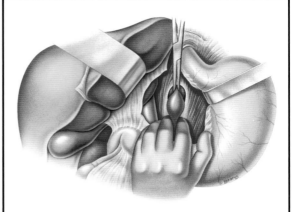

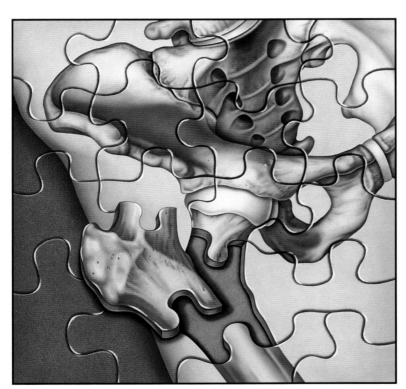

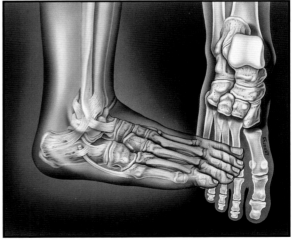

ROBIN LAZARUS
814 Edgewood Drive
Westbury, NY 11590
(516) 338-0636
FAX (516) 334-5105

AREAS OF SPECIALIZATION: Anatomical, surgical and conceptual illustration in full color, halftone or line for textbooks, atlases, posters, journals and advertisements.

CLIENTS: Mosby-Year Book, W.B. Saunders, Doubleday, Cliggott Publishing and several other publishers, private physicians and advertising agencies.

PROFESSIONAL BACKGROUND: B.F.A., Illustration, Syracuse University. M.A., Medical and Biological Illustration, Johns Hopkins School of Medicine.

PROFESSIONAL MEMBERSHIPS: Association of Medical Illustrators, Graphic Artists Guild.

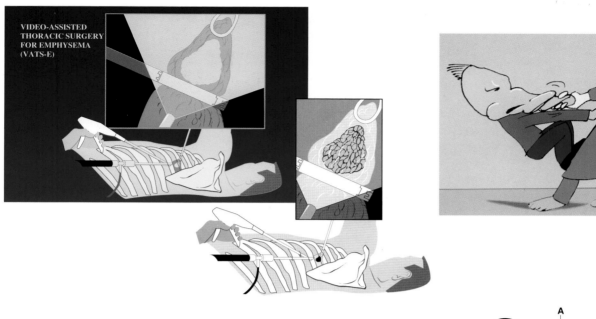

VIDEO-ASSISTED
THORACIC SURGERY
FOR EMPHYSEMA
(VATS-E)

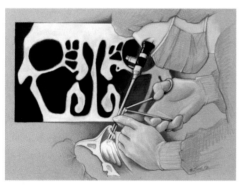

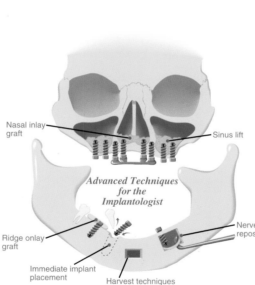

Nasal inlay
graft

Sinus lift

*Advanced Techniques
for the
Implantologist*

Ridge onlay
graft

Nerve
repositioning

Immediate implant
placement

Harvest techniques

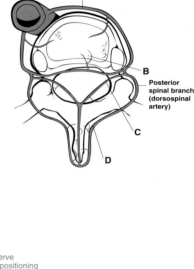

A

B

Posterior
spinal branch
(dorsospinal
artery)

C

D

Level I
Level II
Level III
Level IV
Level V
Level VI

Pam Little, A.M.I.

9878 North Kendall Drive #G110
Miami, Florida 33176
(305)547-6783 work
(305)595-3472 home

Areas of Specialization: Medical, biological and editorial illustration in color and black and white computer and traditional media

Professional Background: Graphics supervisor/Medical Illustrator since 1987 for the University of Miami School of Medicine; M.A. from University of Texas Southwestern Graduate School, 1984

Clients: Medical Marketing Int'l.; W.B. Saunders Publishing Co., Elsevier Science Publishing Co., Jobson Publications

Professional Memberships: Active member, Association of Medical Illustrators; member, Guild of Natural Science Illustrators

MARK LEFKOWITZ

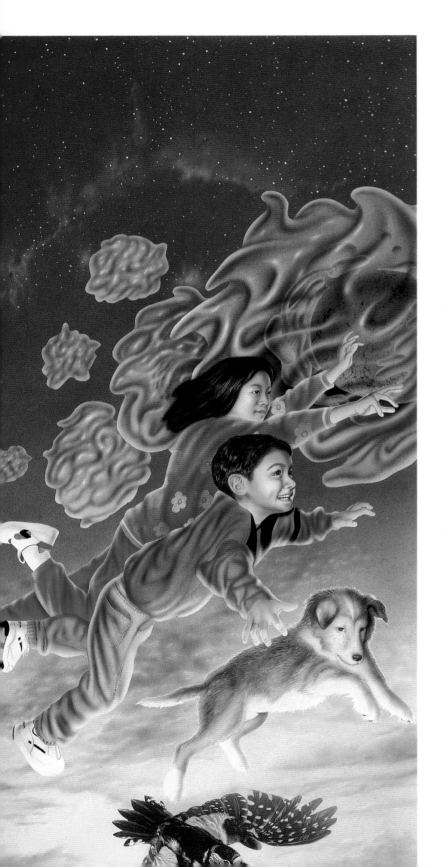

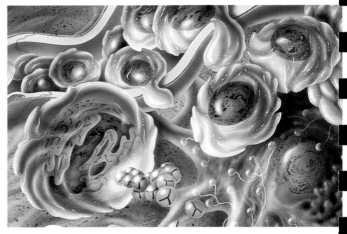

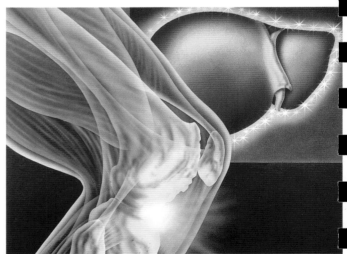

Mark Lefkowitz Associates

Medical and Conceptual
I l l u s t r a t i o n

132 Oak Hill Drive
Sharon, MA 02067
(617) 784-5293
FAX (617) 784-1951

MARK LEFKOWITZ

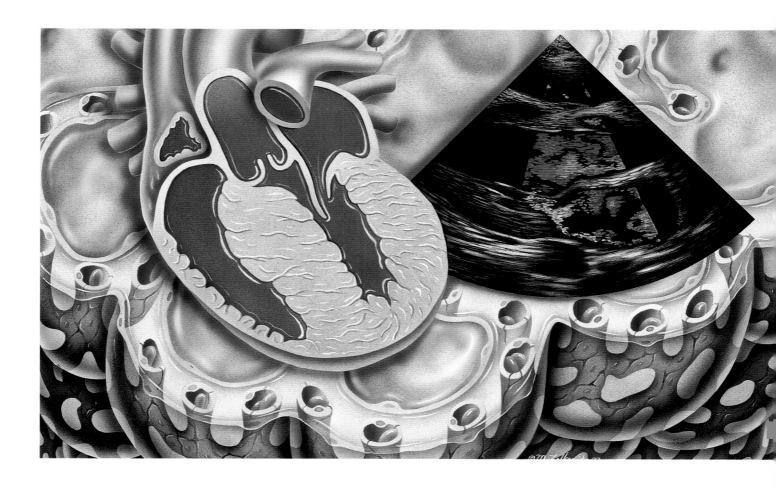

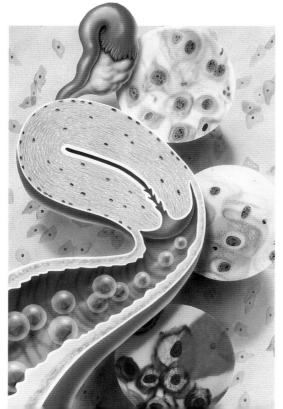

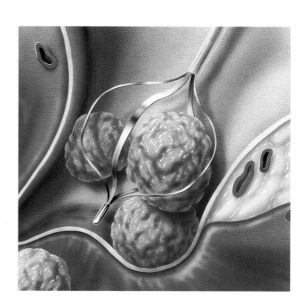

Medical and Conceptual
Illustration
(617) 784-5293

ROBERT MARGULIES
M A R G U L I E S   M E D I C A L   A R T

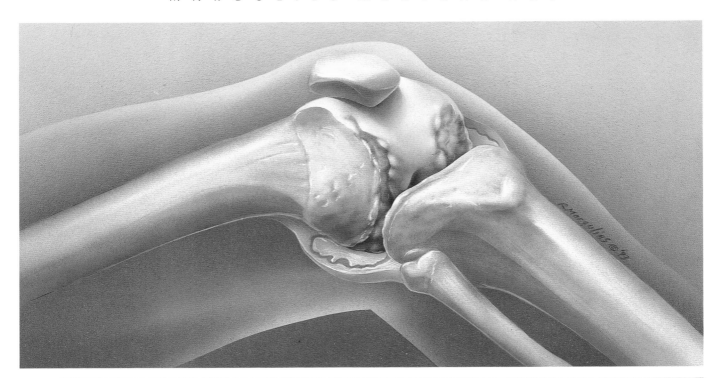

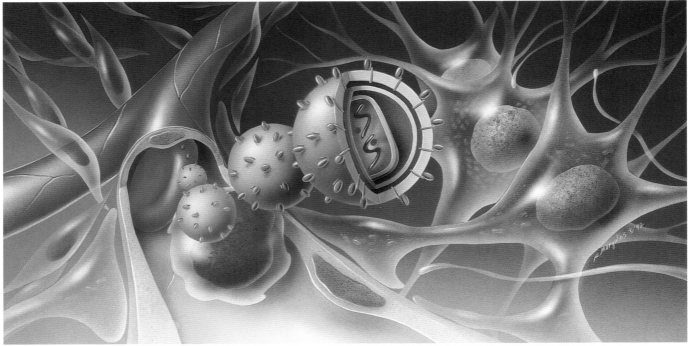

ROBERT MARGULIES

Margulies Medical Art
561 Broadway, 10-B
New York, NY 10012
(212) 219-9621
FAX (212) 334-8459

AREAS OF SPECIALIZATION: Full-color
conceptual illustration for medical publishing
and pharmaceutical advertising. Anatomical and
surgical illustration. Art direction and storyboards for computer animation.

CLIENTS: Pharmaceutical advertising agen-
cies, medical journals and publishers. A
selected list includes: Frank J. Corbett, William
Douglas McAdams, J. Walter Thompson, Cliggott
Publishing Co., Maclean Hunter Medical
Communications.

Animation clients include Pfizer Inc., Lederle
International, and Windsor Digital. Illustrator
for a series of 3-D pop-up books commissioned
by Wyeth Ayerst laboratories.

PROFESSIONAL BACKGROUND: M.S.,
Medical Illustration, Medical College of
Georgia. Four years professional experience
with Duke University Medical Center. Self-
employed since 1982.

PROFESSIONAL MEMBERSHIP:
Association of Medical Illustrators.

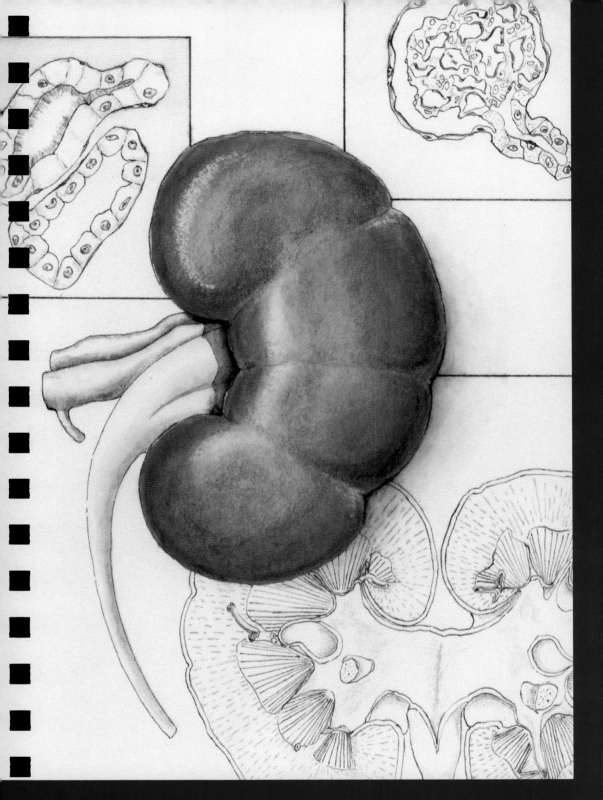
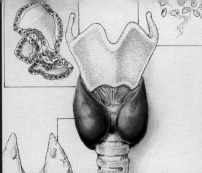
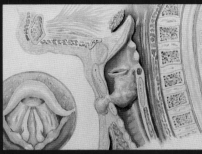
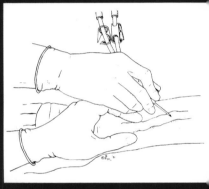
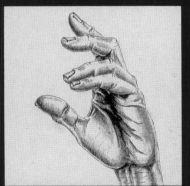
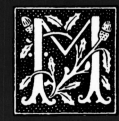

Area of Specialization:

Medical and Scientific illustration for publishing, advertising, and medicolegal purposes.

Media:
Black and White *(pen and ink, graphite and carbon dust)*

Color *(watercolor, pastel dust, pencil, gouache, acrylic)*

Clients Include:

■ Thomas Jefferson Medical School
■ UMDNJ- Rutgers Medical School
■ Polyclinic Hospital, Harrisburg, PA
■ Igaku-Shoin Publishing Company, NY
■ Lankenau Hospital, Philadelphia, PA
■ AKCESS Medical Products Inc., New Brunswick, NJ

Education:

Associate Art Degree, University of the Arts, Philadelphia, PA
Major: Illustration

Doctor of Medicine, Temple University School of Medicine, Philadelphia, PA

Bachelor of Arts, Denison University, Granville, OH
Major: Biology

BETTY MARCHANT, M.D.

7 Killington Court
Old Bridge, NJ 08857
908.679.0017

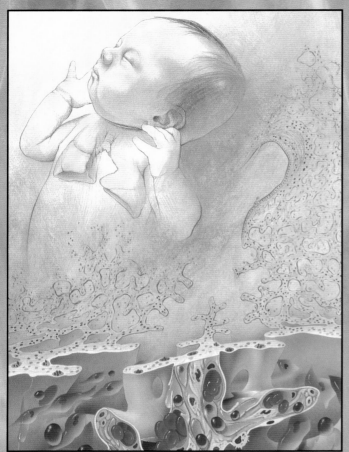
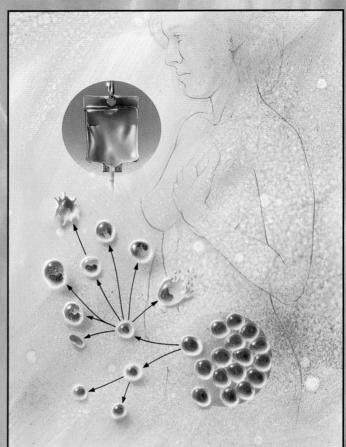
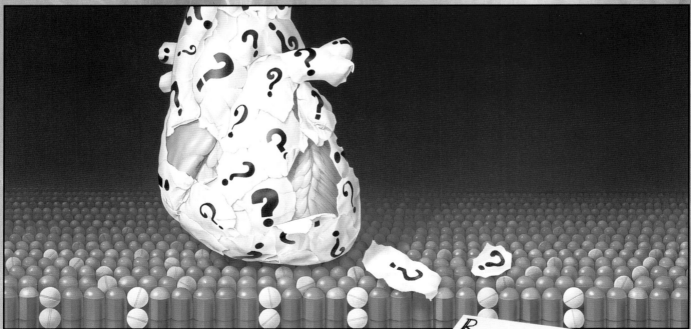

MARTENS & KIEFER

Craig L. Kiefer
Kimberly A. Martens
200 E. 5th Avenue, #420
Naperville, IL 60563
Phone/FAX (708) 355-6590

Eastern Region
Represented by:
Carol Chislovsky Design Inc.
(212) 677-9100   Fax: (212) 353-0954

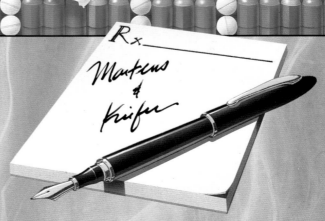

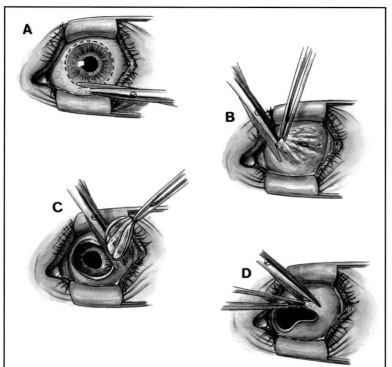

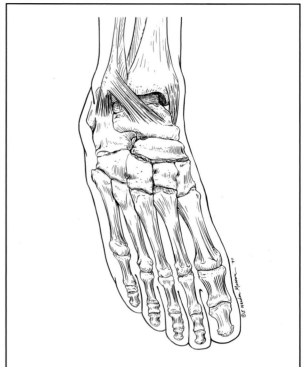

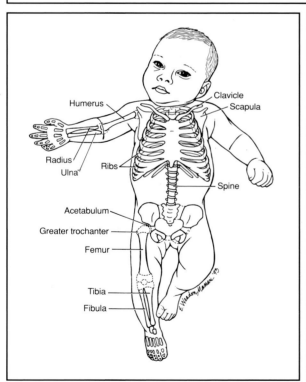

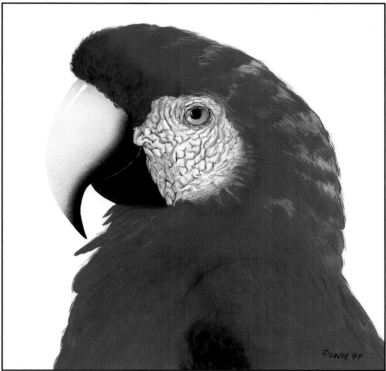

ELIZABETH W. MASSARI, MSMI, CMI

5913 Willoughby Avenue
Los Angeles, CA 90038
Phone/FAX (213) 461-3833
(800) 400-3833

AREAS OF SPECIALIZATION: Anatomical, surgical, medical/dental product and natural science subjects rendered in line, tone and color with traditional media and computer. Illustration and graphic services for publication, projection media, courtroom and exhibit/display.

CLIENTS: Mosby-Year Book, Simon and Schuster, McGraw-Hill, J.B. Lippincott, Churchill-Livingstone, Raven Press, NICU Ink, March of Dimes, Philips Interactive Media, Merck, Gen-Probe, Core-Vent/Dentsply, Urological Sciences Research Foundation, Body Integration Chiropractics, Advanced Surgical Intervention, numerous medical journals, private physicians, health professionals and attorneys, UCLA Medi-cal Center, Kaiser Permanente, Olive View Medical Center, Cedars Sinai Medical Center.

PROFESSIONAL BACKGROUND: Master of Science in Medical Illustration, Medical College of Georgia. B.A. in Art/Biology, Judson College. Full-time freelance illustrator and graphic artist.

PROFESSIONAL MEMBERSHIPS: Association of Medical Illustrators, Guild of Natural Science Illustrators, Women in Design of Los Angeles, Society of Illustrators of Los Angeles.

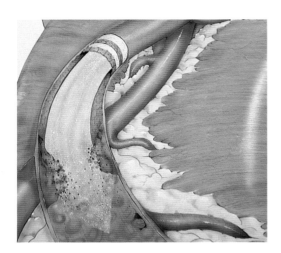

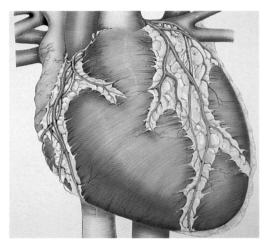

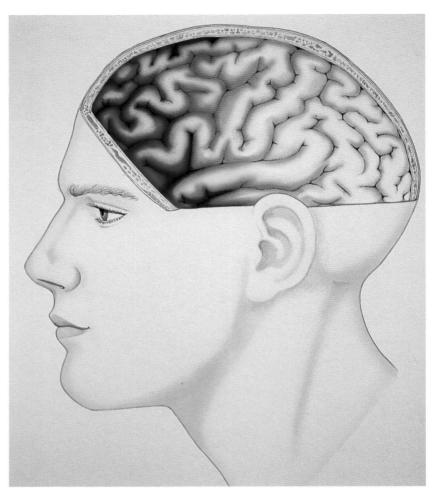

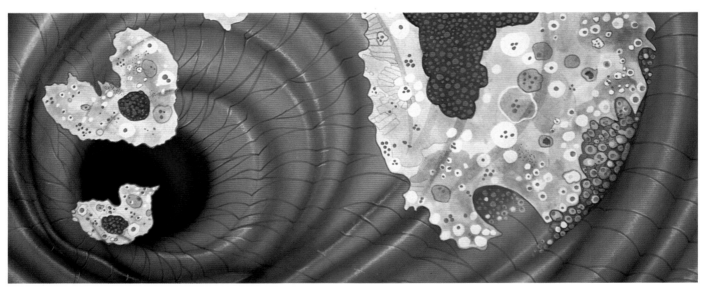

LAWRENCE MAY
Illustrator
6430 Lincoln Road
Bradenton, FL 34203
(813) 751-6536

AREAS OF SPECIALIZATION:
Cardiology
Electrophysiology
Metaphysical Healing

CLIENTS:
Electrocatheter Corporation
E.P. Technologies, Inc.
Visualizations for Health, Llewellyn Publishing
Memorial Hospital, Sarasota, Florida
The U.S. Army

PROFESSIONAL BACKGROUND:
B.F.A.
Registered Nurse, CCRN, CEN.

PROFESSIONAL MEMBERSHIPS:
Association of Medical Illustrators.

OTHER: 18D Special Forces Medical NCO.

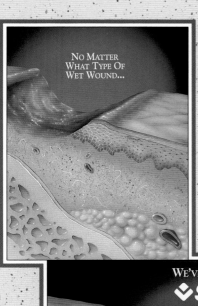

NO MATTER
WHAT TYPE OF
WET WOUND...

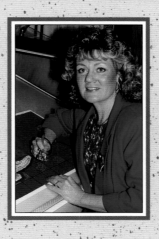

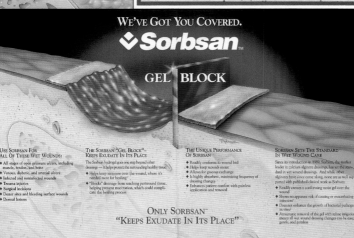

WE'VE GOT YOU COVERED.

❖ Sorbsan™

GEL BLOCK

USE SORBSAN FOR ALL OF THESE WET WOUNDS:
- ◆ All stages of open pressure ulcers, including muscle, tendon, and bone
- ◆ Venous, diabetic, and arterial ulcers
- ◆ Infected and noninfected wounds
- ◆ Trauma injuries
- ◆ Surgical incisions
- ◆ Donor sites and bleeding surface wounds
- ◆ Dermal lesions

THE SORBSAN "GEL BLOCK"— KEEPS EXUDATE IN ITS PLACE
The Sorbsan hydrogel goes one step beyond other dressings — it helps protect the surrounding healthy tissue.
- ◆ Helps keep moisture over the wound, when it's needed most for healing
- ◆ "Blocks" drainage from reaching periwound tissue, helping prevent maceration, which could complicate the healing process

THE UNIQUE PERFORMANCE OF SORBSAN
- ◆ Readily conforms to wound bed
- ◆ Helps keep wounds moist
- ◆ Allows for gaseous exchange
- ◆ Is highly absorbent, minimizing frequency of dressing changes
- ◆ Enhances patient comfort with painless applicaton and removal

SORBSAN SETS THE STANDARD IN WET WOUND CARE
Since its introduction in 1989, Sorbsan, the market leader in calcium alginate dressings, has set the standard in wet wound dressings. And while other alginates have since come along, none are as well supported with published clinical work as Sorbsan.
- ◆ Readily creates a conforming moist gel over the wound
- ◆ Shows no apparent risk if causing or exacerbating infection
- ◆ Does not enhance the growth of bacterial pathogens in vitro
- ◆ Atraumatic removal of the gel with saline irrigation means all wet wound dressing changes can be easy, gentle, and painless

ONLY SORBSAN™
"KEEPS EXUDATE IN ITS PLACE"

The keys to success and a steady work flow in today's economy are versatility and flexibility, not only in style and technique, but also in choosing clientele and marketplaces in which to generate business. Medical art is inherently specialized, because the subject matter areas one illustrates are medical, biological or scientific. As a sole proprietor in medical illustration, my goal is to consistently maintain quality and craftsmanship, but to adapt the look and feeling of my work to harmonize with a wide variety of marketplaces, audiences, and usage.

An illustration's message, what it **says**, is just as important as its method, **how it says what it says**. The emotion it elicits from the viewer may be dark and dramatic, texturally exciting, technically intricate or soft and fuzzy. I adjust my palette and technique to meet the requirements of the assignment. If given full artistic license, I paint the feelings conveyed by a verbal description or by the words in an author's story.

Medical content and accuracy are paramount to medical illustration. But sometimes intentional departures and exaggerations of reality for drama and emphasis may also be an integral part of an artistic endeavor. Whether you react to the combination of colors, the textures and contrasts, or identify with the subject matter itself, my illustrations are intended to stimulate a response. It is my hope that these works will inspire you in some way.

—*Current Trends and Versatile Imagery:
The Medical Art of Teri McDermott
International Museum of Surgical Science, Chicago
One person show: Spring, 1994*

TERI J. McDERMOTT, MA CMI

38W563 KOSHARE TRAIL

ELGIN, ILLINOIS 60123

TEL: 708 ◆ 888 ◆ 2206

FAX: 708 ◆ 888 ◆ 2210

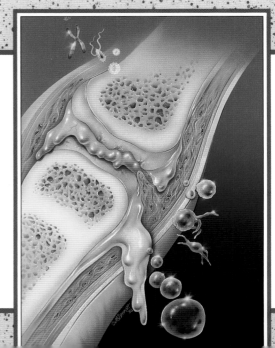

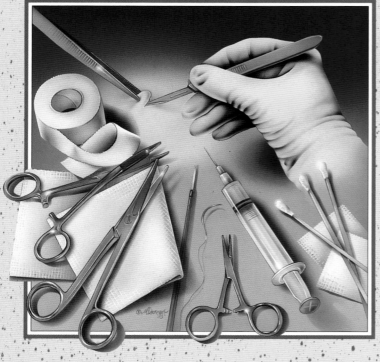

TERI J. McDERMOTT, MA CMI

38W563 KOSHARE TRAIL

ELGIN, ILLINOIS 60123

TEL: 708♦888♦2206

FAX: 708♦888♦2210

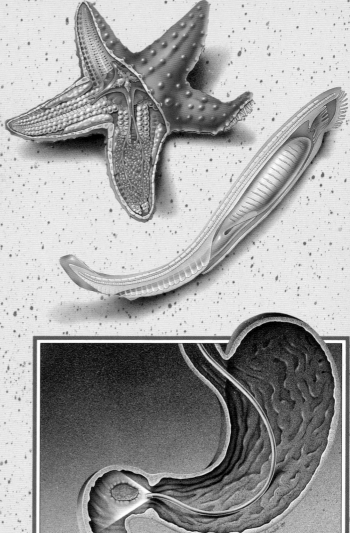

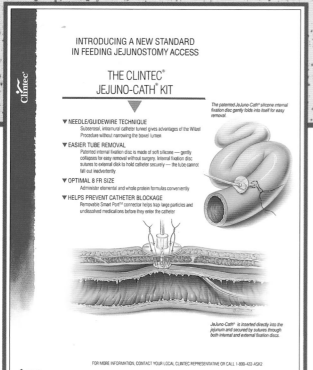

INTRODUCING A NEW STANDARD
IN FEEDING JEJUNOSTOMY ACCESS

THE CLINTEC®
JEJUNO-CATH® KIT

▼ NEEDLE/GUIDEWIRE TECHNIQUE
Subserosal, intramural catheter tunnel gives advantages of the Witzel
Procedure without narrowing the bowel lumen

▼ EASIER TUBE REMOVAL
Patented internal fixation disc is made of soft silicone — gently
collapses for easy removal without surgery. Internal fixation disc
sutures to external disk to hold catheter securely — the tube cannot
fall out inadvertently

▼ OPTIMAL 8 FR SIZE
Administer elemental and whole protein formulas conveniently

▼ HELPS PREVENT CATHETER BLOCKAGE
Removable Smart Port™ connector helps trap large particles and
undissolved medications before they enter the catheter

The patented JeJuno-Cath® silicone internal
fixation disc gently folds into itself for easy
removal.

JeJuno-Cath® is inserted directly into the
jejunum and secured by sutures through
both internal and external fixation discs.

FOR MORE INFORMATION, CONTACT YOUR LOCAL CLINTEC REPRESENTATIVE OR CALL 1-800-422-ASK2

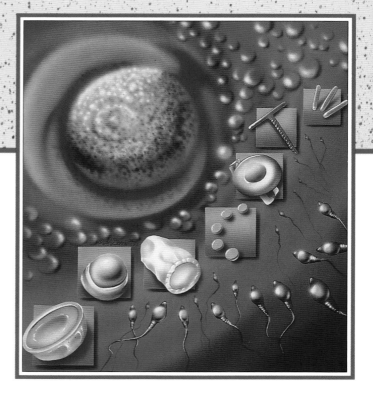

TERI J. McDERMOTT, MA CMI

38W563 KOSHARE TRAIL

ELGIN, ILLINOIS 60123

TEL: 708 ♦ 888 ♦ 2206

FAX: 708 ♦ 888 ♦ 2210

*M*aster of Arts in Instructional Design with High Honors from the University of Missouri. Bachelor of Science in Medical art with Honors from the University of Illinois.

Board Certified Medical Illustrator with nineteen years of professional experience. Full time freelance practice since 1981, serving clients nationwide and overseas.

Winner of 23 awards from the Association of Medical Illustrators, Graphic Design: USA, and New York's Rx Club. Work included in **The Best in Medical Advertising and Graphics**, vols. I & II, and in exhibitions at Chicago's International Museum of Surgical Science and Museum of Science & Industry, the Rochester Institute of Technology, and elsewhere in the US, Australia and Great Britain.

President, Association of Medical Illustrators, 1994-95.

Time or economic restrictions?
An extensive file of stock art is available for reuse. Please call with your request for existing imagery to fulfill your most urgent requirements.

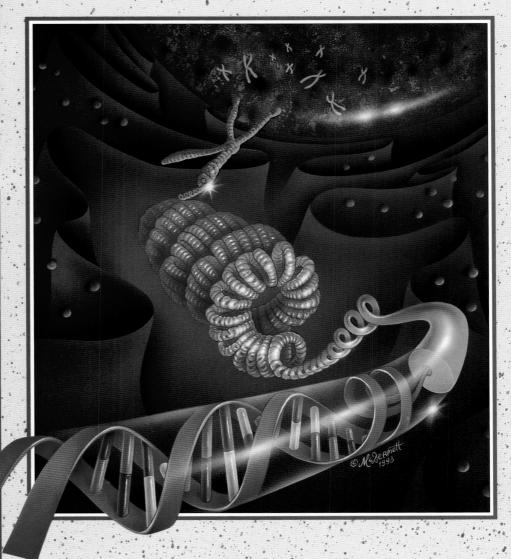

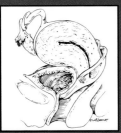

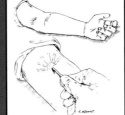

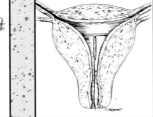

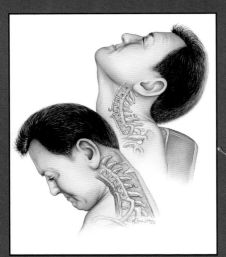

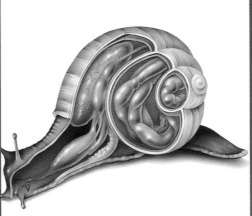

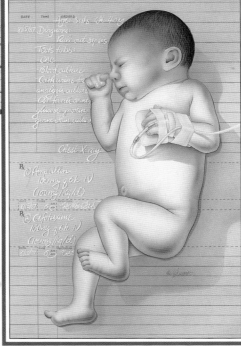

PAGE DESIGN BY PAT SURBELLA

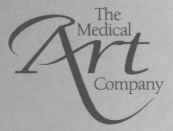

The Medical Art Company

Quality Standards
• Clear, concise images
• Scientific accuracy
• Elegant, colorful style
• On-time delivery

Contact Marcia Hartsock, CMI
2142 Alpine Place
Cincinnati, Ohio 45206-2603
TEL 513 221-3868
FAX 513 221-3859

National Clients
• Churchill Livingstone, Inc.
• Krames Communications
• Marion Merrell Dow
• Medical Economics Publishers
• Ortho Pharmaceuticals
• Procter & Gamble
• W.C. Brown Publishers
• Williams & Wilkins

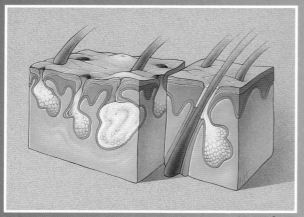

Acne Vulgaris

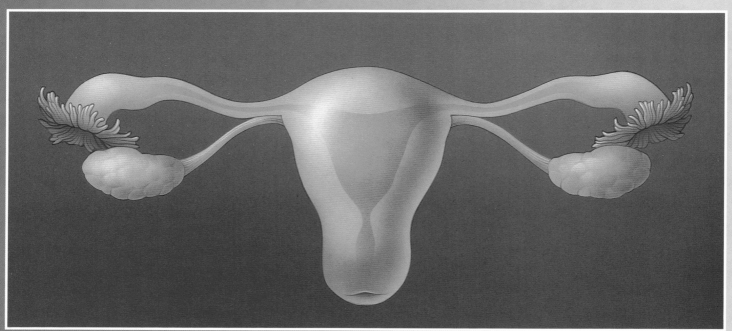

Female Reproductive Organs

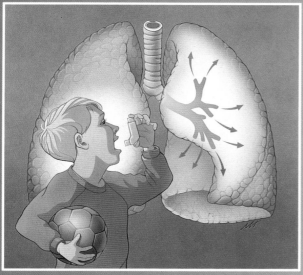

Inhalation Therapy

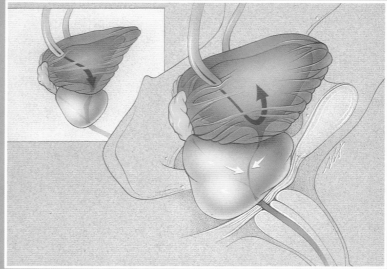

Prostatitis

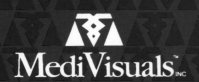

MediVisuals INC

Thomas D. Sims, President
1221 River Bend Dr., Ste. 240
Dallas, Texas 75247

4050 Innslake Dr., Ste. 200
Glen Allen, Virginia 23060

(214) 634-3996 • (800) 899-2154
Fax (214) 634-7947

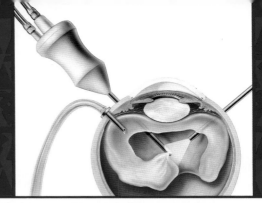

- *Medical/Pharmaceutical Advertising*
- *Textbook/Journal Illustration*
- *Editorial Illustration*
- *Medical-legal*
- *Animation*
- *Models*

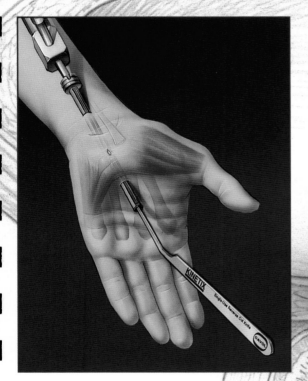

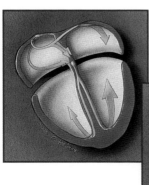

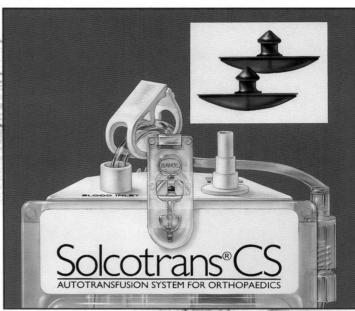

Solcotrans® CS
AUTOTRANSFUSION SYSTEM FOR ORTHOPAEDICS

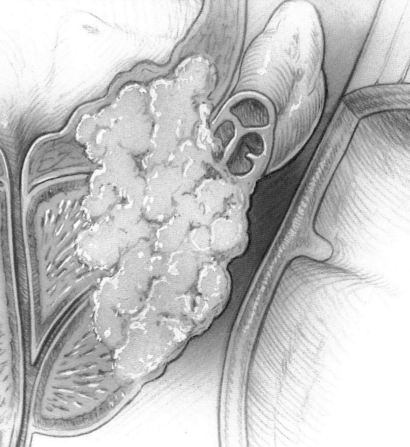

Greater depth and speed of learning, increased retention, and deeper understanding of complex material are the hallmarks of multimedia communications.

MedPro Communications, Inc., a licensed developer for A.D.A.M. Software, specializes in content-based, interactive, multimedia products for the pharmaceutical, health-care, and legal industries.

With an experienced team of medical illustrators, medical and technical writers, programmers, and production specialists, MedPro builds upon the extraordinary A.D.A.M. database of medical illustrations. Our deliverables include user-driven, portable marketing programs, sales training modules for in-house and field use, diskettes as direct-mail and giveaways, patient education programs, and interactive kiosks. Our media and platforms are as varied as our clients, including laserdisc, CDI, CD-ROM, diskette, videotape, and print.

A.D.A.M. Software, Inc. (Animated Dissection of Anatomy for Medicine), is an internationally-recognized Georgia-based company that creates, publishes, and markets multimedia software based on human anatomy. The A.D.A.M. database includes over six thousand precisely rendered, richly detailed illustrations from every layer of the human body, as well as libraries of physiology, histology, radiology, pathology, and surgery.

For more information about MedPro, please contact Catherine Twomey, President, or John Yesko at (708) 831-0911.

Med|Pro
Communications, Inc.

1360 Old Skokie Road
Suite 2 S.W.
Highland Park, IL 60035

Phone (708) 831-0911
Fax (708) 831-0980

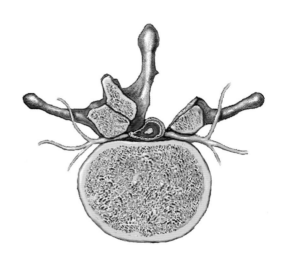

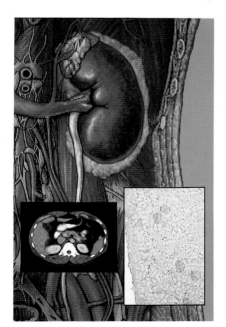

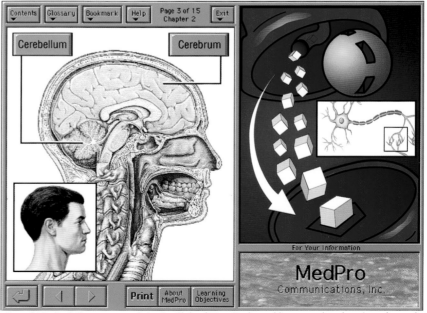

MedPro has won Awards of Excellence from the Association of Medical Illustrators and the Rx Club of New York, and has completed projects for such clients as Pfizer Pharmaceuticals, Lederle Pharmaceuticals, Fujisawa, and Abbott Labs.

Fran Milner

3300 Longview Drive
San Bruno, CA 94066
(415) 355 7984

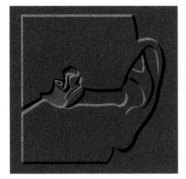

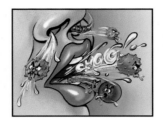

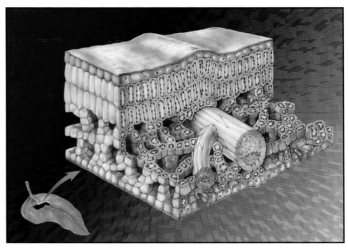

Computer Generated
Medical and
Biological Illustrations

All images on this
page were created
digitally.

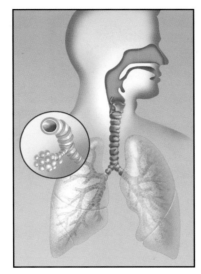

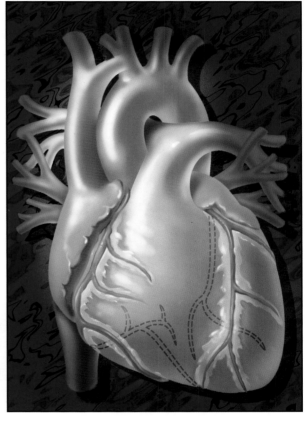

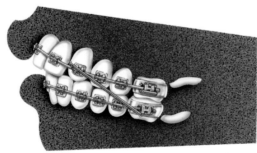

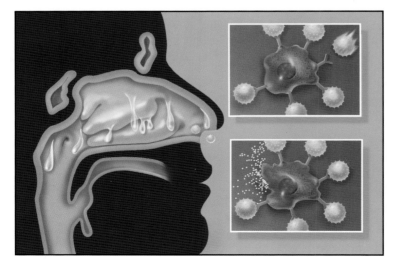

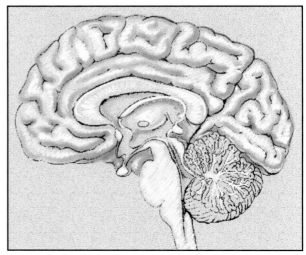

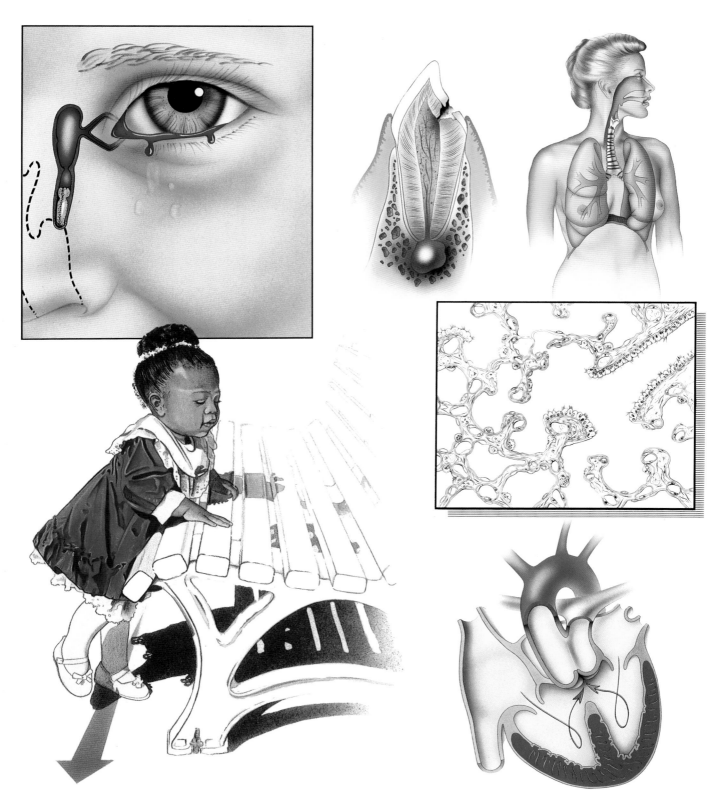

BRIAR LEE MITCHELL, MA
11552 Hartsook Street
Valley Village, CA 91601
(818) 752-6809
FAX (818) 752-8043

AREAS OF SPECIALIZATION: Book illustration (brush/pen & ink, 2 colour, tone or full colour). Illustration and animation for video, film or print. Medical/legal. Cel-vinyl. Posters.

CLIENTS: The Annenberg Centre for Health Sciences, AT&T, Burroughs Wellcome, Coca-Cola, Disney, Genentech, Inc., Good Housekeeping, Harvard Medical Library, Hearst Books, International Masters Publications, John Wiley, Inc., Johns Hopkins Medical Institutions, Lifetime Medical Television, Lucasfilm, Ltd., MacMillan Publishing, McDonald's, Reader's Digest, The Smithsonian, Subak-Sharpe Communications, William Morrow & Co., Yale Medical School.

PROFESSIONAL BACKGROUND: Master of Art in Medical and Biological Illustration. Medical Illustrator since 1977. Internships with the Arizona Heart Institute and The Annenberg Centre for Health Sciences.

PROFESSIONAL MEMBERSHIPS: Association of Medical Illustrators, Society of Illustrators of Los Angeles.

AWARDS/HONORS: Gold Key award for interactive computer program, art and story boards, 1989; Second Place, Projection Media, AMI Salon, 1987; John Muir Film Festival, art and animation for video production, 1985.

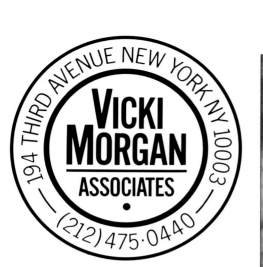

VICKI MORGAN ASSOCIATES

194 THIRD AVENUE NEW YORK NY 10003

(212) 475·0440

REPRESENTING HEALTHCARE ILLUSTRATORS

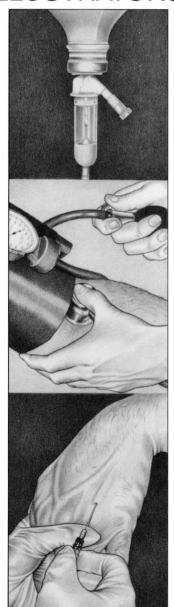

WENDY WRAY

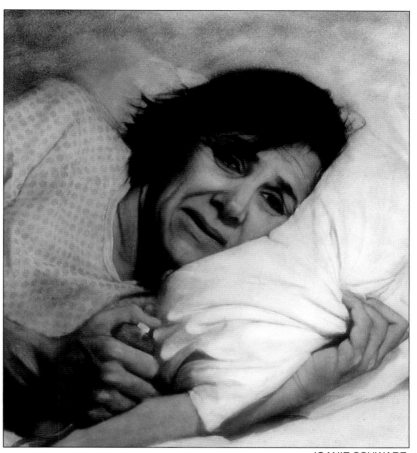

JOANIE SCHWARZ

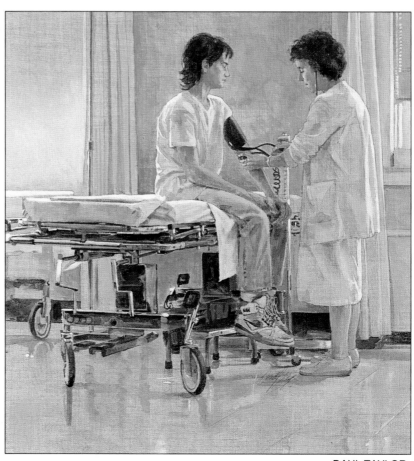

DAHL TAYLOR

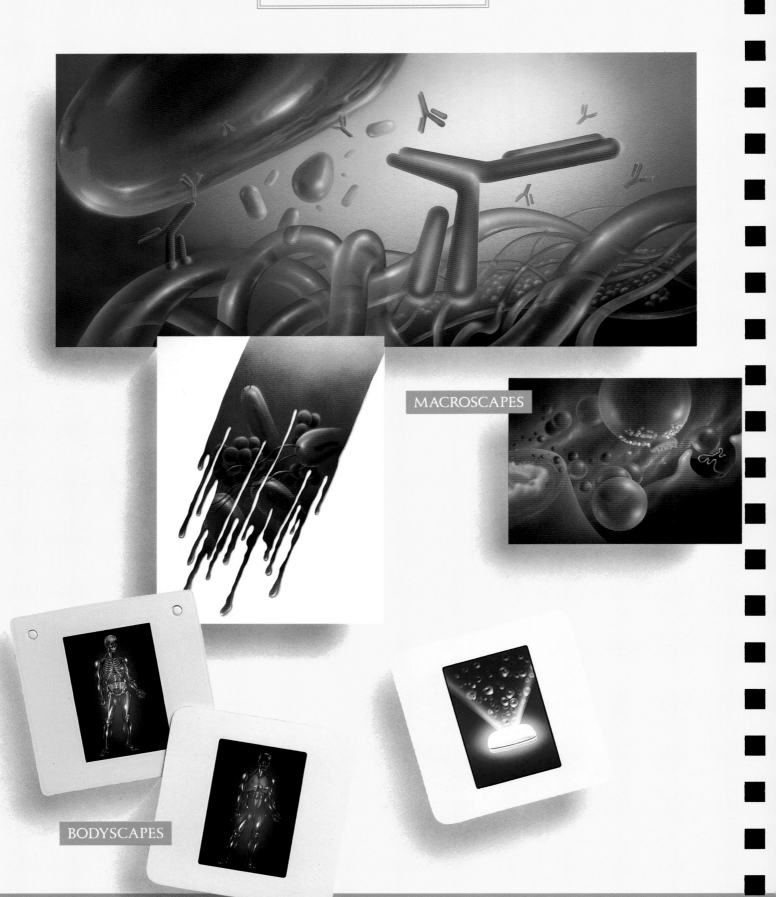

MACROSCAPES

BODYSCAPES

GALERIE D'ART

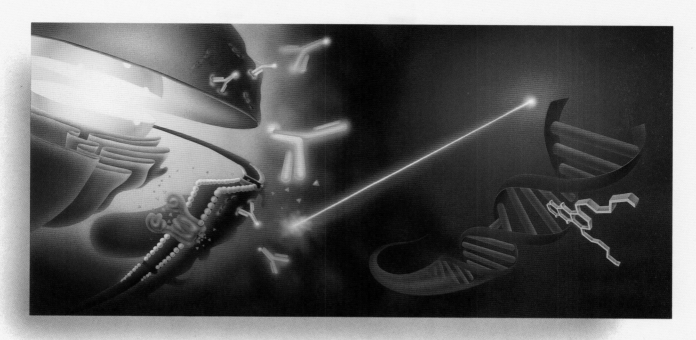

CELLULAR PORTRAITS

Medical Illustration

1116 Elm Street
Peekskill, New York
10566
914 736-7823

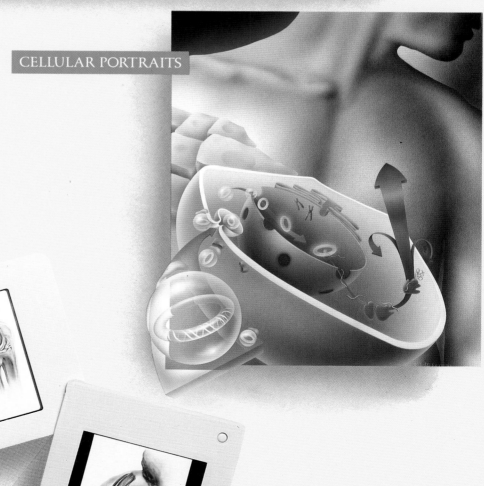

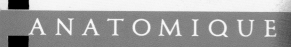

ANATOMIQUE

LEONARD MORGAN

MEDICAL ART

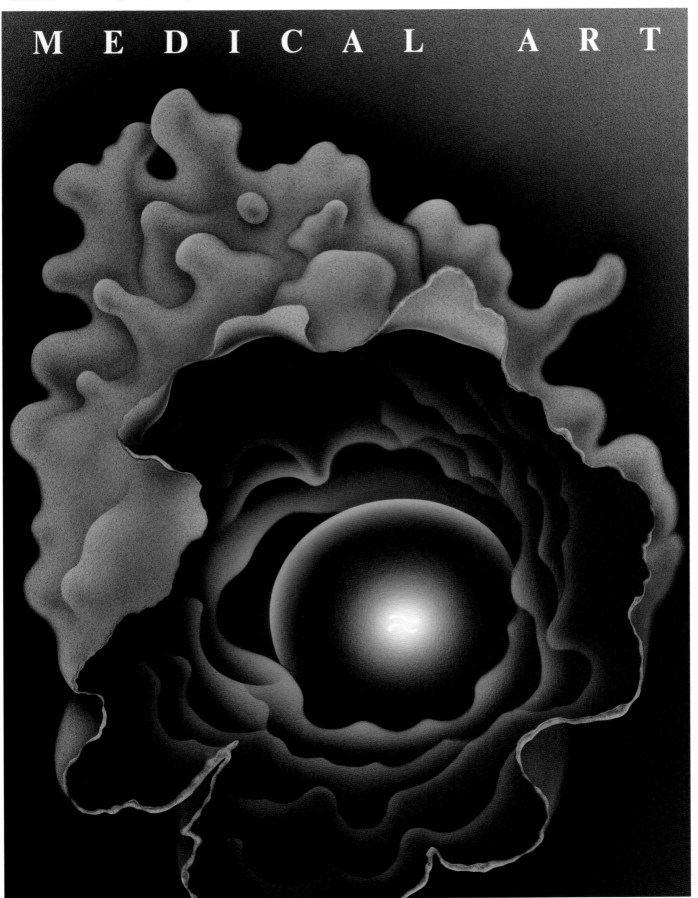

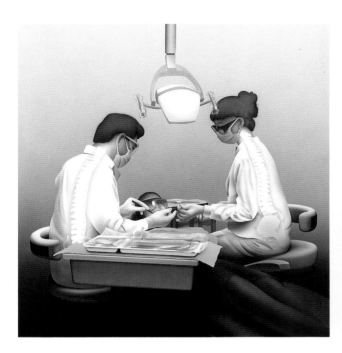

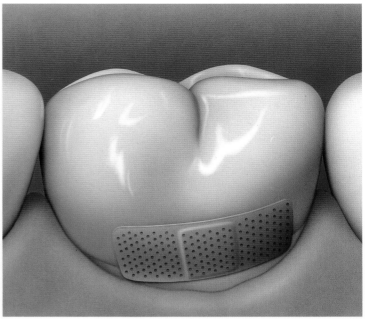

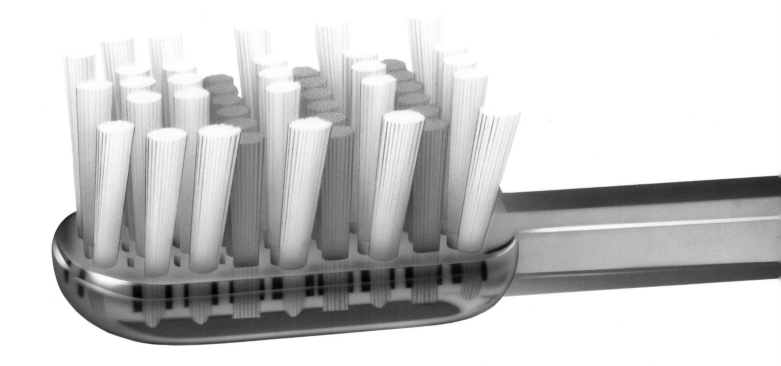

LEONARD E. MORGAN, INC.

730 Victoria Court
Bolingbrook, Illinois 60440
(708) 739-7705
FAX (708) 739-1885

PROFESSIONAL BACKGROUND: BOARD
CERTIFIED MEDICAL ILLUSTRATOR with 18
years full-time professional freelance experience serving clients coast to coast. Bachelor's
Degree, Medical Art, 1974, University of Illinois
at the Medical Center in Chicago.

AREAS OF SPECIALIZATION: Medical
advertising art, medical product illustration,
high tech imaging, dental illustration, editorial
covers, anatomy, biology, geology, and space art.

PROFESSIONAL MEMBERSHIPS: Association of Medical Illustrators, Midwest Medical
Illustrators Association.

AWARDS/HONORS: Inclusion in the Rx Club
Show 1992, 1990, 1989, 1988, 1987; *The Best in
Medical Advertising and Graphics, 1989*; ADDY

AWARD 1988; *Prints Regional Design Annual*,
1989, 1987, 1985; Society of Illustrators Show,
Art of Medicine, 1987; The One Show, 1987;
Communications Arts Advertising Annual,
1987; *Illustration Annual*, 1986, 1985; International Show of Medical Art in Milan, Italy, 1986.

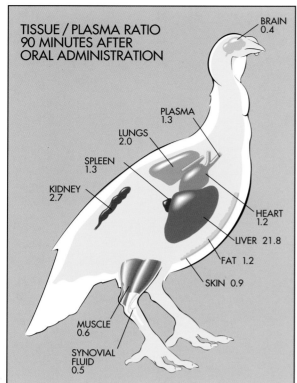

TISSUE / PLASMA RATIO
90 MINUTES AFTER
ORAL ADMINISTRATION

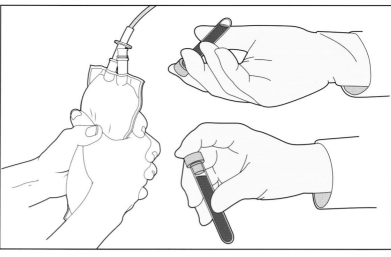

Reproduction of Illustration from AxSym Operations Manual has been granted with approval of Abbott Laboratories, all rights reserved by Abbott Laboratories.

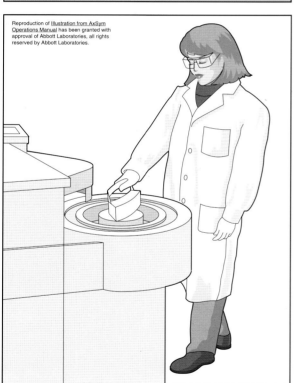

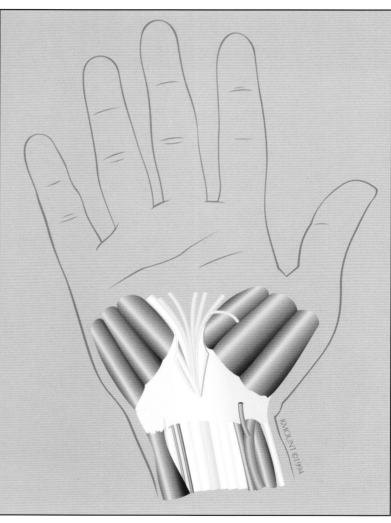

KRISTIN MOUNT

Computer Generated Medical Imagery
4356 N. Bell Avenue, I-3
Chicago, IL 60618
(312) 539-9311

AREAS OF SPECIALIZATION: Computer generated medical illustration in line, tone, and color for advertising and publishing use. Specialize in figures, hands, surgical instruments, and hospital products.

CLIENTS: Abbott Laboratories, TAP Pharmaceuticals, Baxter Healthcare Corporation, Lutheran General Hospital, Product Communications, Inc.

PROFESSIONAL BACKGROUND: M.A.M.S. in Medical Illustration, University of Illinois at Chicago.

PROFESSIONAL MEMBERSHIPS: Association of Medical Illustrators.

AWARDS/HONORS: 1992 Vesalian Scholar. Featured slide set artist at the 1992 SIGGRAPH Computer Graphics Conference.

OTHER: Also experienced in preparation of art for film, including trapping, choking and color separation.

KeelinMurphy

BFA MAMS MEDICAL ILLUSTRATION

(516) 689-5435

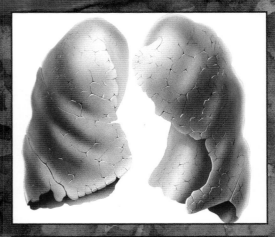

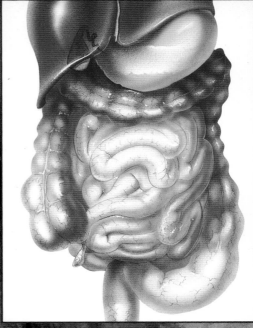

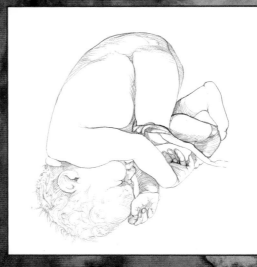

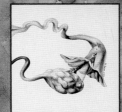

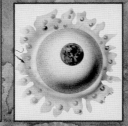

NEW YORK WEST
MEDICAL ILLUSTRATION STUDIO

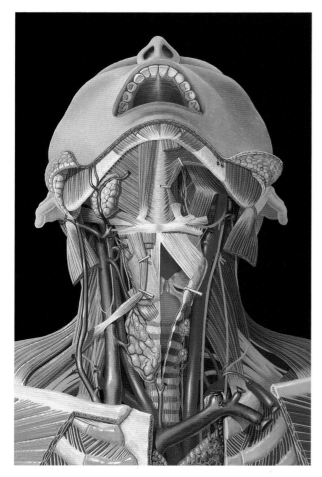
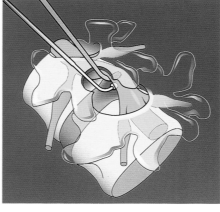
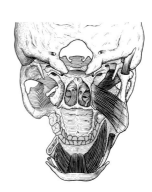
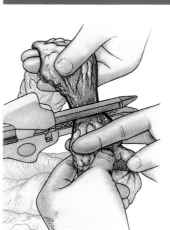
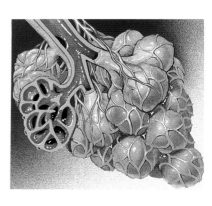
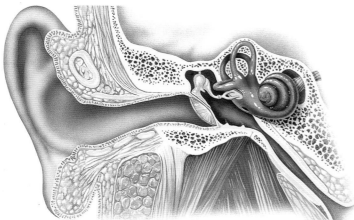
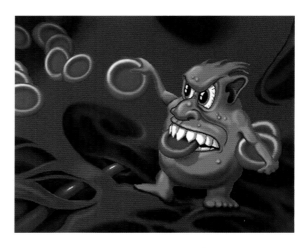

DAVID R. PURNELL, M.A., C.M.I.
New York West
P.O. Box 260
Lonsdale, MN 55046
Phone/FAX (507) 744-5408

AREAS OF SPECIALIZATION: Clearly-demonstrated surgical concepts and procedures rendered as 3-D video animation or still art for publication. Particular application to teaching institutions and medical device manufacturers.

SPECIAL INTEREST: Graphic support of medical research into the body's electromagnetic substructure; body/mind/spirit relationship to health and disease.

PROFESSIONAL BACKGROUND: Memorial Sloan-Kettering Cancer Center, New York City—chief medical/surgical illustrator, 1974–1992. Routinely worked beside surgeons in the operating room.

M.A. degree in Medical Illustration, The Johns Hopkins University School of Medicine, 1973. In 1993, David Purnell opened NEW YORK WEST Medical Illustration Studio near Minneapolis, Minnesota.

PROFESSIONAL MEMBERSHIPS: Association of Medical Illustrators.

STEVE OH

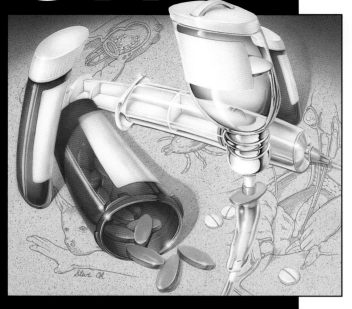

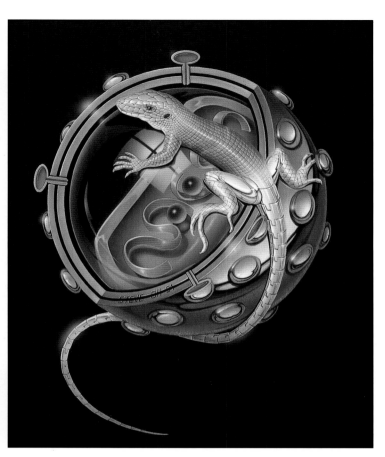

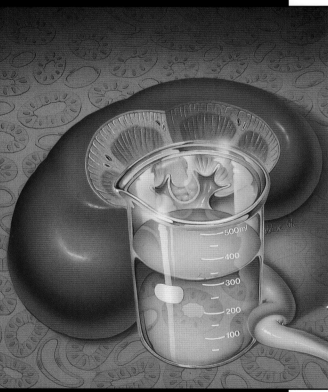

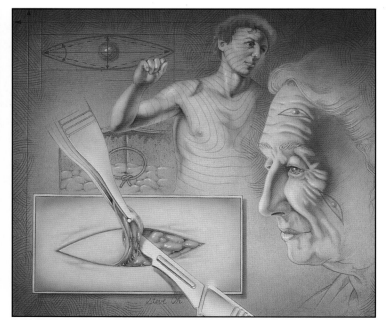

Steve Oh, M.S.
STUDI-OH Medical Art
4901 McWillie Circle, No. 232
Jackson, Mississippi 39206
Telephone and FAX (601) 366-6470

153

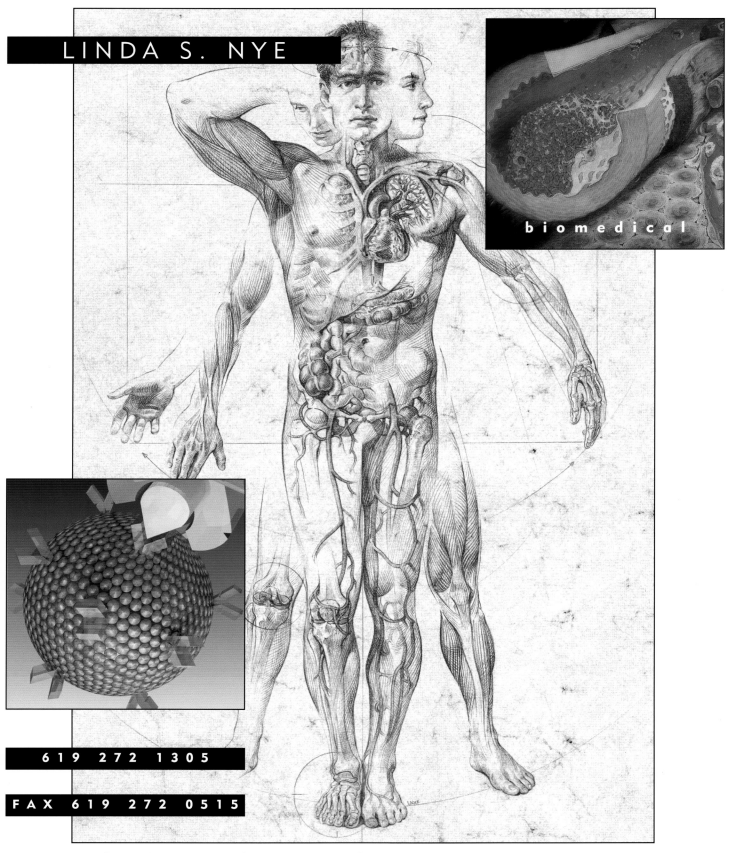

LINDA S. NYE

biomedical

619 272 1305

FAX 619 272 0515

Specializing in biomedical, scientific, and anatomical art for corporate communications and advertising.
All media including, Macintosh based computer illustration, and 3D modeling.

Clients include: Hybritech, Baxter, Allergan, Gensia, Weekly Reader, Advanced Tissue Sciences, Quidel,
Corvas, Cytel, Amylin, Immune Response Corp., Mentus, Inc.

Member: Society of Illustrators, AMI, IAAA

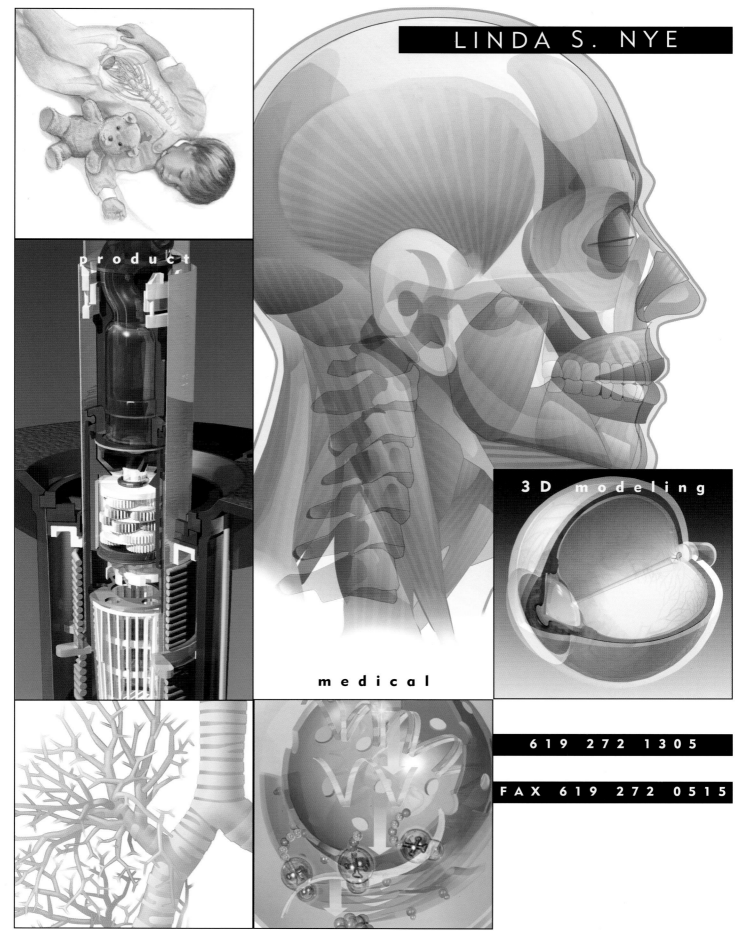

LINDA S. NYE

product

3D modeling

medical

619 272 1305

FAX 619 272 0515

155

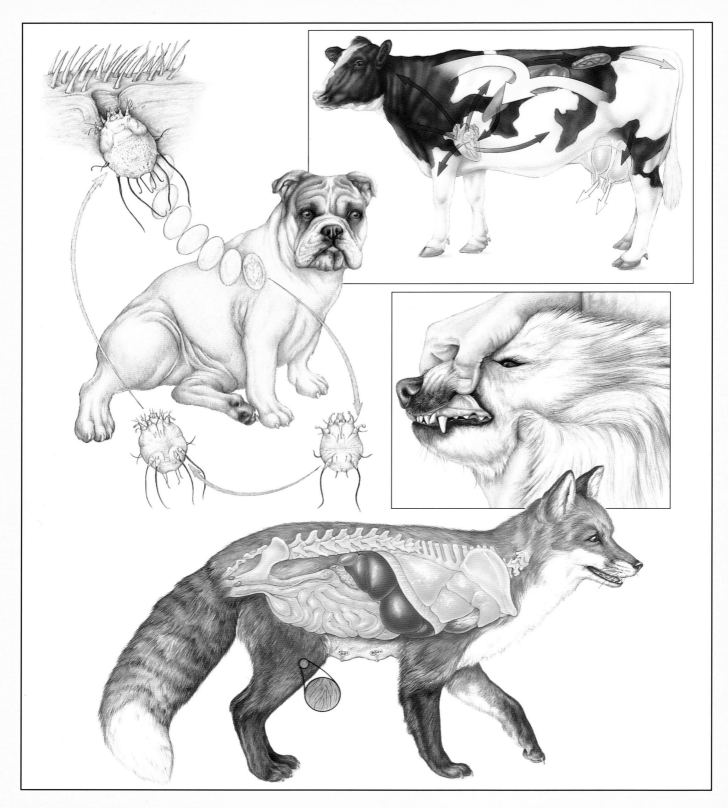

LAURIE O'KEEFE
30096 Kennedy Gulch Road
Conifer, CO 80433
(303) 838-5966

Specializing in textbook illustration for all educational levels, veterinary, and pharmaceutical product visuals.

CLIENTS: Editorial and textbook publishers, medical product companies, physicians, and environmental organizations. A selected list includes: Addison Wesley, Benjamin/Cummings, DC Heath, FOCA, Glencoe/McGraw-Hill, Johnson Hill Press, Scott Foresman, Tim Peters & Co., West Pub., Wm. C. Brown, Veterinary Medicine Pub.

PROFESSIONAL BACKGROUND:
B.S. Zoology
M.S. Anatomy/Medical Illustration
Colorado State University

PROFESSIONAL MEMBERSHIPS: Association of Medical Illustrators, Guild of Natural Science Illustrators.

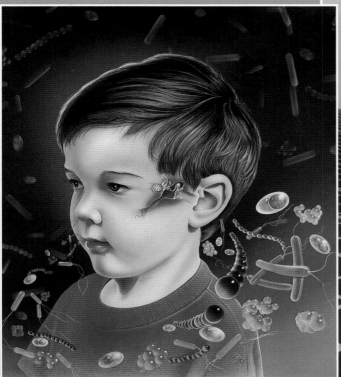

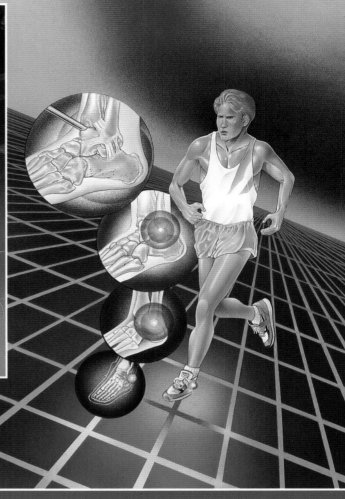

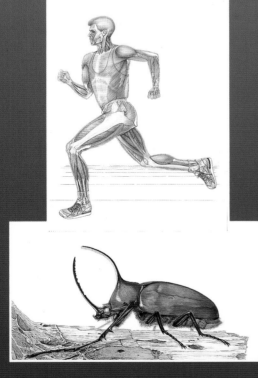

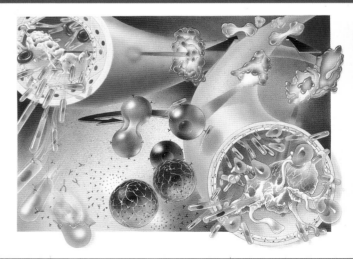

FELIPE PASSALACQUA, C.M.I.

WBI Worldwide Biomedic Images
401 Cedar St.
San Antonio, TX 78210
(210) 226-1718
FAX (210) 226-1640

AREAS OF SPECIALIZATION: Medical, scientific, editorial and medical legal illustrations executed in airbrush, acrylics, tone and line in a dynamic, creative, understandable and accurate manner.

PROFESSIONAL BACKGROUND: B.S., Sacred Heart University, P.R., Post Baccalaureate degree in Medical Illustration, Ohio State University.

PROFESSIONAL MEMBERSHIPS: Association of Medical Illustrators, Guild of Natural Science Illustrators, Midwest Medical Illustrators.

AWARDS/HONORS: Best of Show and Honorable Mention at AMI Midwest Regional Meeting 1993.

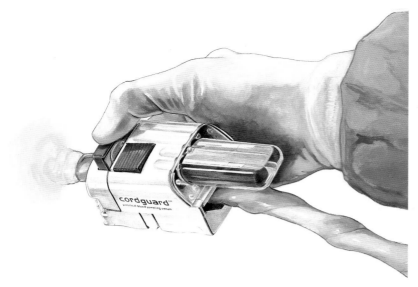

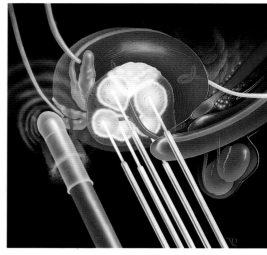

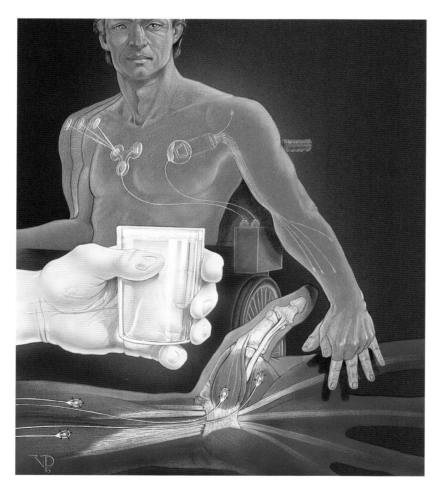

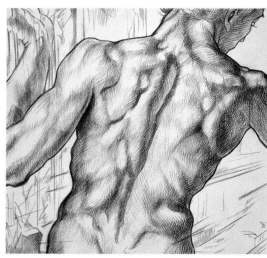

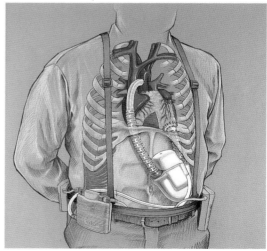

VINCENT PEREZ STUDIO

Vincent Perez
1279 Weber Street
Alameda, CA 94501
(510) 521-2262
FAX (510) 522-2300

AREAS OF SPECIALIZATION: Medical, Editorial and Fantasy Illustration; Paintings; Drawings; Pop-Ups and Woodcuts.

CLIENTS (partial list): Syntex, Immunex, *Time* Magazine, National Medical Enterprises, Cutter Labs, LucasFilm, ABC-TV, Disney, Hana Biologics, Hewlett-Packard, CIBA-GEIGY; *RN* Magazine; Oral B; Science.

PROFESSIONAL BACKGROUND (partial list): BFA, Pratt Institute, NY, 1960; MFA, CA College of Arts & Crafts, 1965; Demonstrating Illustrator at the APLAR Meeting, Bali, Indonesia; ILAR Meeting, Barcelona, Spain and the AAOS, New Orleans, LA.

PROFESSIONAL MEMBERSHIPS:
GAG, SISF, AMI.

AWARDS/HONORS (partial list): Gold–Rx Club, Western Art Director's Club; Excellence–LULU, Print, CA, Mead, In-Awe; Merit–SINY, AIGA, SILA, RX.

OTHER: See also: *American Showcase 9, 10, 11, 12; Bay Area Creative Sourcebook 1 & 2; LA Workbook 12, '92 & '94; Creative Illustration 1; GAG Directory 7, 8, 9; Medical Illustration Sourcebook 4, 5, 6.*

158

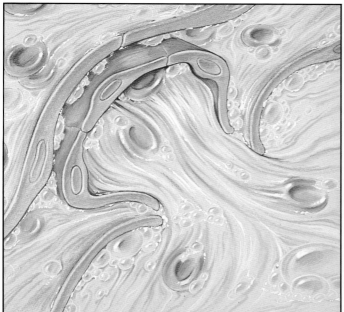
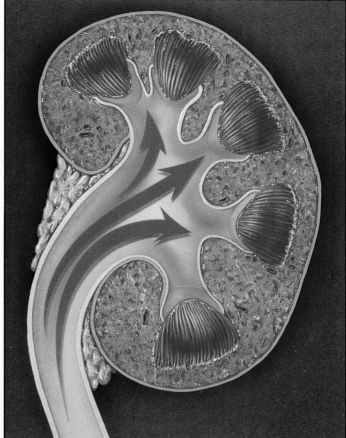
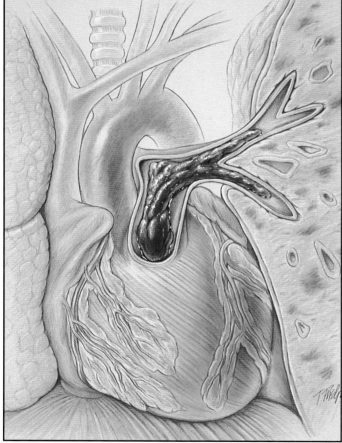
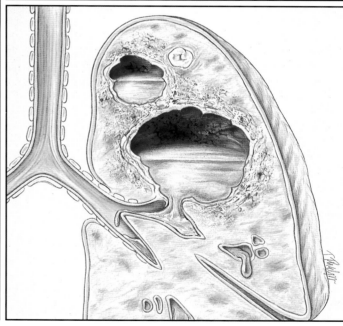

TIM PHELPS, CMI, FAMI

504 Fairway Court
Towson, Maryland 21286
(410) 955-3213   (410) 321-8607

AREAS OF SPECIALIZATION: Creative and concise solutions to anatomical, biological, conceptual and surgical illustration problems in full color, pen and ink, tone and computer for clients nationwide.

PROFESSIONAL BACKGROUND: Certified Medical Illustrator, M.S., Medical and Biological Illustration, University of Michigan. Associate Professor, Johns Hopkins, Fellow in Association of Medical Illustrators. Fourteen years professional experience specializing in editorial and publishing markets.

SELECTED CLIENTS:

Book Publishers: Elsevier, Lea & Febiger, JB Lippincott, Little Brown & Co., Mosby-Yearbook, The Quarasan Group, Raven Press, W.B. Saunders, Springer-Verlag, Williams and Wilkins, Worldbook Encyclopedia.

Editorial: ABC News, American Family Physician, Anatomyworks, BioLiterature, *Cricket* Magazine for Children, *The Houston Post, Medical Economics, Medical Times*, NBC News, *Postgraduate Medicine*.

Advertising: Adams/Sandler Group, AM Medica, Becton-Dickinson, Medical Information Services, Miller-Mauro Group, Ogilvy-Mather, Parke-Davis, Warner-Lambert.

OTHER: Over 30 awards in national and regional markets.

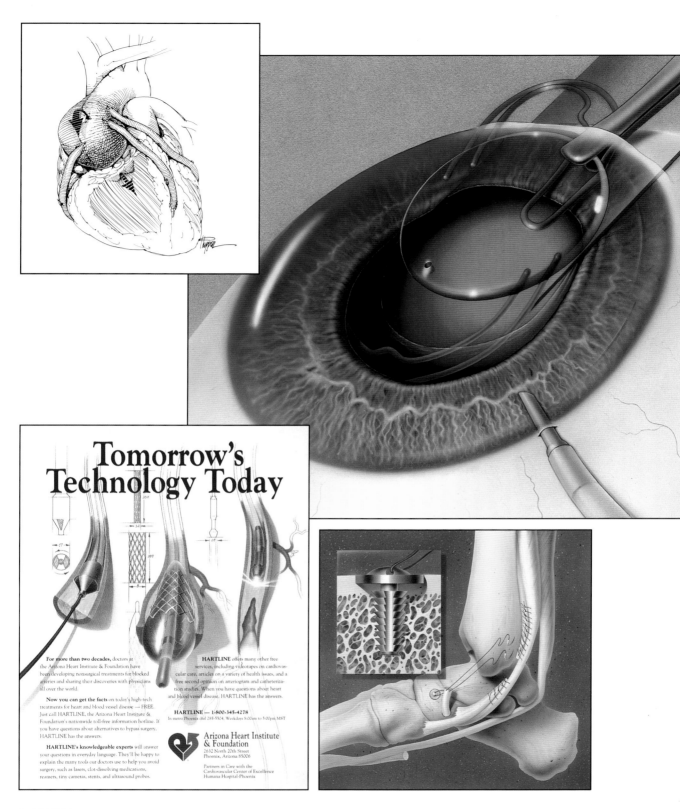

Tomorrow's
Technology Today

For more than two decades, doctors at the Arizona Heart Institute & Foundation have been developing nonsurgical treatments for blocked arteries and sharing their discoveries with physicians all over the world.

Now you can get the facts on today's high-tech treatments for heart and blood vessel disease — FREE. Just call HARTLINE, the Arizona Heart Institute & Foundation's nationwide toll-free information hotline. If you have questions about alternatives to bypass surgery, HARTLINE has the answers.

HARTLINE's knowledgeable experts will answer your questions in everyday language. They'll be happy to explain the many tools our doctors use to help you avoid surgery, such as lasers, clot-dissolving medications, reamers, tiny cameras, stents, and ultrasound probes.

HARTLINE offers many other free services, including videotapes on cardiovascular care, articles on a variety of health issues, and a free second opinion on arteriogram and catheterization studies. When you have questions about heart and blood vessel disease, HARTLINE has the answers.

HARTLINE — 1-800-345-4278
In metro Phoenix dial 285-5304. Weekdays 8:00am to 5:00pm MST

Arizona Heart Institute & Foundation
2632 North 20th Street
Phoenix, Arizona 85006

Partners in Care with the
Cardiovascular Center of Excellence
Humana Hospital-Phoenix

SPENCER PHIPPEN

14014 North 32nd St. #152
Phoenix, AZ 85032
(602) 482-7863

AREAS OF SPECIALIZATION: Conceptual, surgical, and anatomical illustrations in color and black & white for advertising and publication.

PROFESSIONAL BACKGROUND: A certified medical illustrator with a Master of Fine Arts in medical illustration from the University of Michigan and over eight years of illustrating experience.

PROFESSIONAL MEMBERSHIPS:
Association of Medical Illustrators.

AWARDS/HONORS: Recipient of a number of national awards including a Certificate of Merit in Advertising Illustration (1992) and a First Place in Projection Media (1990) from the Association of Medical Illustrators.

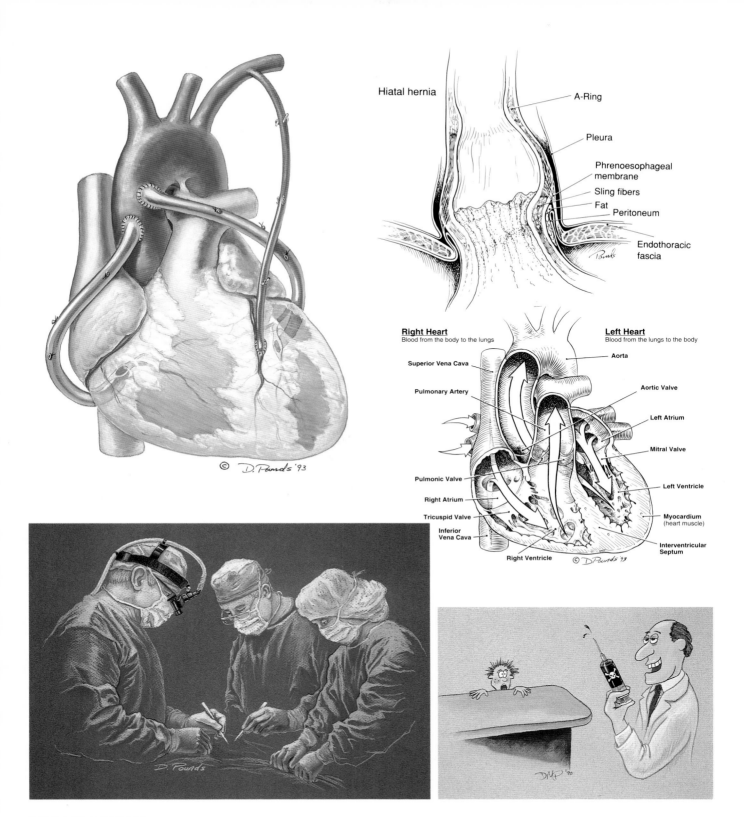

Hiatal hernia

A-Ring

Pleura

Phrenoesophageal membrane

Sling fibers

Fat

Peritoneum

Endothoracic fascia

Right Heart
Blood from the body to the lungs

Left Heart
Blood from the lungs to the body

Superior Vena Cava

Aorta

Pulmonary Artery

Aortic Valve

Left Atrium

Mitral Valve

Left Ventricle

Pulmonic Valve

Right Atrium

Tricuspid Valve

Inferior Vena Cava

Myocardium (heart muscle)

Interventricular Septum

Right Ventricle

© D Pounds '93

DAVID M. POUNDS

D. Pounds Illustration
1102 Melrose Street
Winston-Salem, NC 27103-4437
Phone/FAX (910) 723-1237

- Conceptualization and visual problem solving; anatomical and surgical illustration for a wide variety of medical specialties produced in all media, both traditional and electronic.

- MA in Biomedical Communications from The University of Texas Southwestern Medical Center.

- Certified medical illustrator and Fellow of the Association of Medical Illustrators.

- Over sixteen years experience in biomedical illustration and communications at the Bowman Gray School of Medicine of Wake Forest University; currently working full time freelance.

161

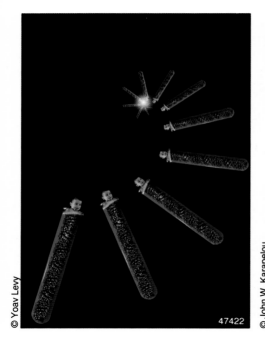

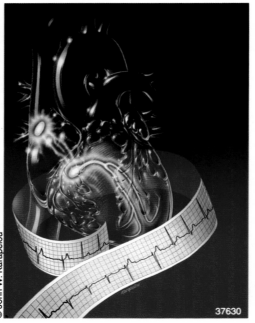

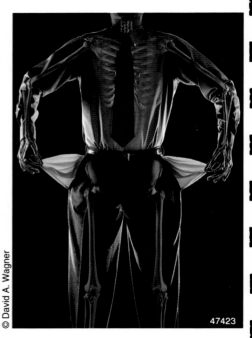

-PHOTOTAKE-

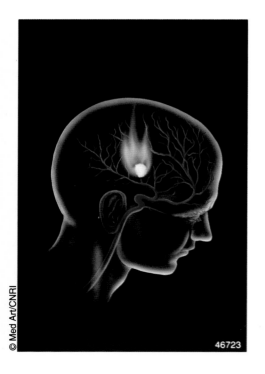

Your Biomedical Stock source when quality matters.

No initial research fee !

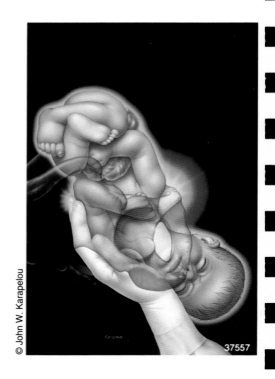

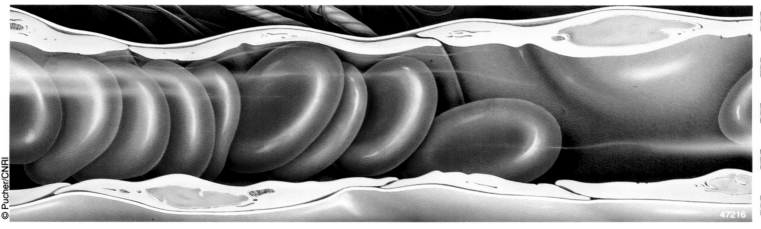

224 West 29th St, New York, NY 10001

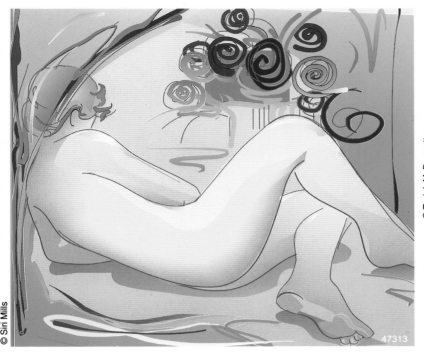
© Siri Mills
47313

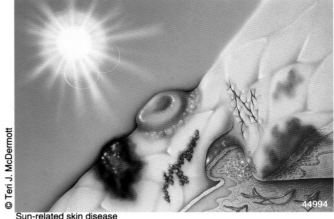
© Teri J. McDermott
Sun-related skin disease
44994

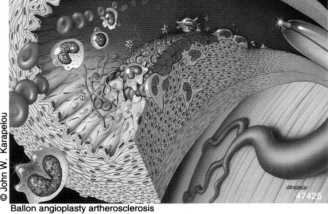
© John W. Karapelou
Ballon angioplasty artherosclerosis
47425

Call for free catalog

800-542-3686

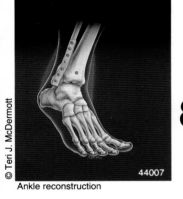
© Teri J. McDermott
Ankle reconstruction
44007

- Vast collection
- 370 Scientific sources
- 24 Worldwide offices

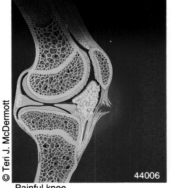
© Teri J. McDermott
Painful knee
44006

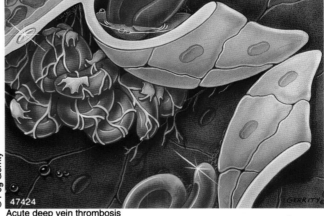
© Peg Gerrity
Acute deep vein thrombosis
47424

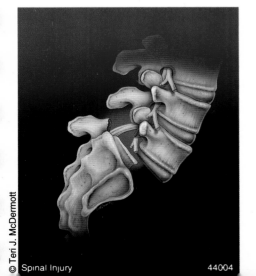
© Teri J. McDermott
Spinal Injury
44004

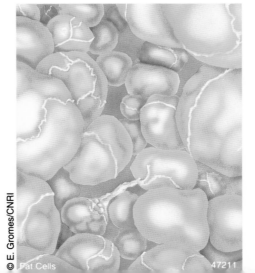
© E. Gromes/CNRI
Fat Cells
47211

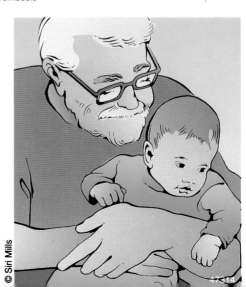
© Siri Mills
47314

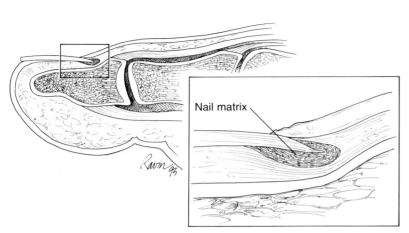

Nail matrix

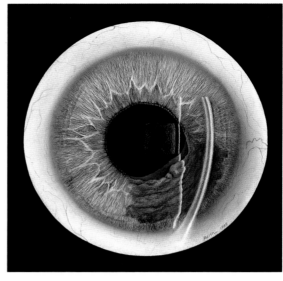

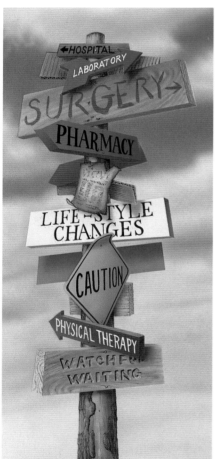

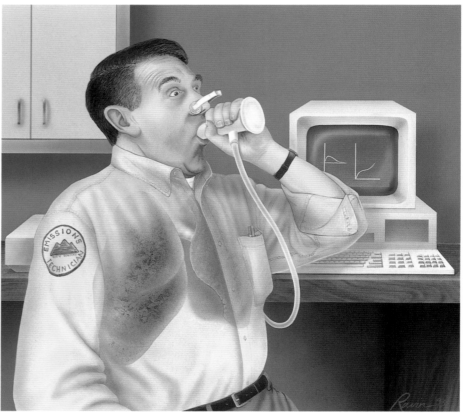

DEBORAH A. RAVIN, C.M.I.

Ravin Art & Design
3253 East Vogel Avenue
Phoenix, Arizona 85028
(602) 494-7752

AREAS OF SPECIALIZATION: Medical and biological illustration in full color, line, and tone for editorial publications, medical and scientific textbooks, advertising, and patient education.

CLIENTS: Include McGraw-Hill Healthcare Publications, Medical Economics Publishing, Raven Press, Ltd., private hospitals, physicians, and attorneys.

PROFESSIONAL BACKGROUND: M.F.A., Medical and Biological Illustration from The University of Michigan; B.F.A., Illustration from Rhode Island School of Design; B.S., Biology and Art from Allegheny College.

PROFESSIONAL MEMBERSHIPS:
Certified member of the Association of Medical Illustrators; Member, Guild of Natural Science Illustrators.

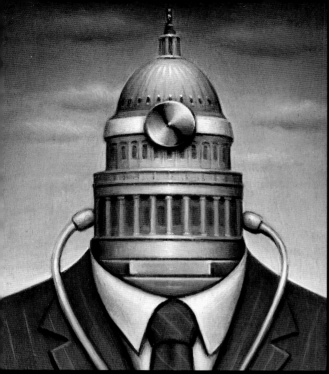
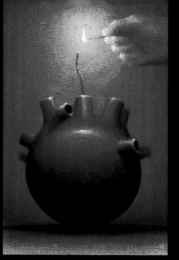
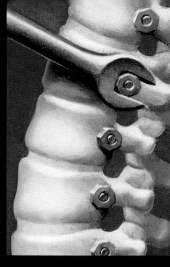
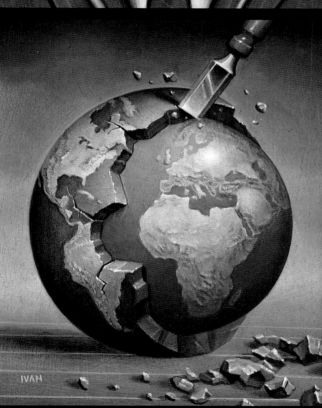
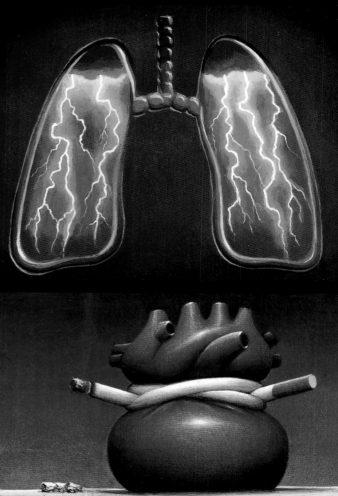

IVAN

VAN SANFORD

310 East 89th Street, #10
New York, NY 10128
(212) 996-9284

AREAS OF SPECIALIZATION: Creative conceptual solutions delivered in full color or continuous tone. Serving editorial, advertising, educational and CGI markets.

CLIENTS: The KSF Group (serving such clients as Lever Brothers, Pfizer International,

Smithkline Beecham, et al.); The McMahon Group (*Anesthesiology News, Gastroenterology and Endoscopy News, General Surgery and Laparoscopy News, Pharmacy Practice News*, et al.); Slack, Inc. (*Journal of Psychosocial Nursing, Orthopedics Today, Gerontological Nursing*, et al.); *Medical Economics*; General Learning Corporation; *Healthcare Forum*; *Medical World News*, Equal Opportunity Publications, Inc.; Viking-Penguin; Economist Intelligence Unit; Risk Management; Associated Press; Kirschenbaum & Bond; Fred Alan

PROFESSIONAL BACKGROUND: B.F.A., Illustration, School of Visual Arts; eight years experience freelance illustrator.

PROFESSIONAL MEMBERSHIPS: Association of Medical Illustrators.

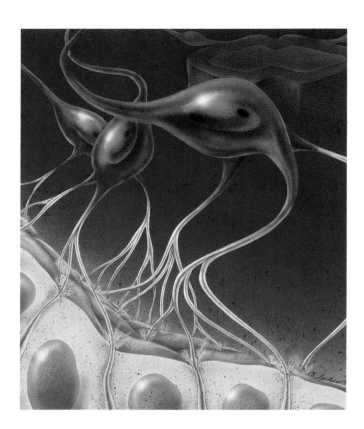
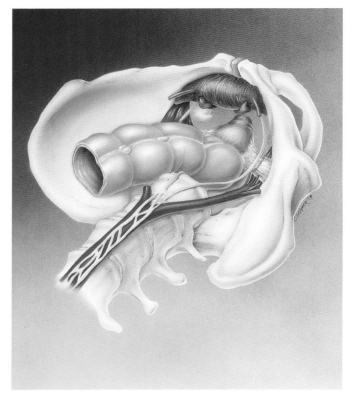
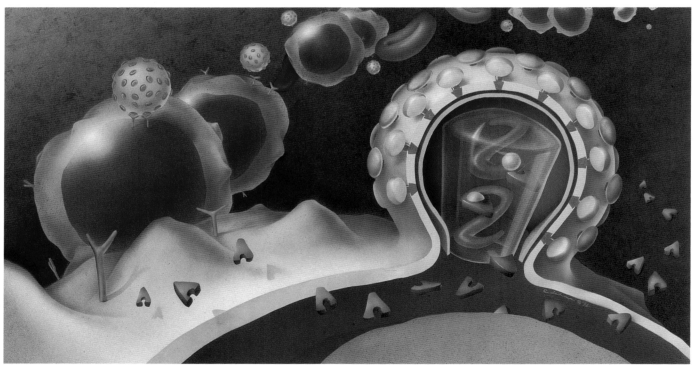

CHRISTINE SCHAAR

330 East 11th Street, Apt. 7
New York, NY 10003
(212) 477-4855
FAX (212) 639-2612

AREAS OF SPECIALIZATION: Full color and B/W conceptual and anatomical illustrations for advertising, editorial, and textbook publication.

CLIENTS: Medical Economics Publishing, J.B. Lippincott Company, Mosby Year Book, Memorial Sloan Kettering Cancer Center, MRI-EFI Publications, and various private physicians.

PROFESSIONAL BACKGROUND: Masters of Associated Medical Sciences, University of Illinois at Chicago. BFA, Illustration, Parsons School of Design.

PROFESSIONAL MEMBERSHIPS: Association of Medical Illustrators

AWARDS/HONORS:
Award of Excellence, Rx Club, 1993
Award of Excellence, AMI, 1993

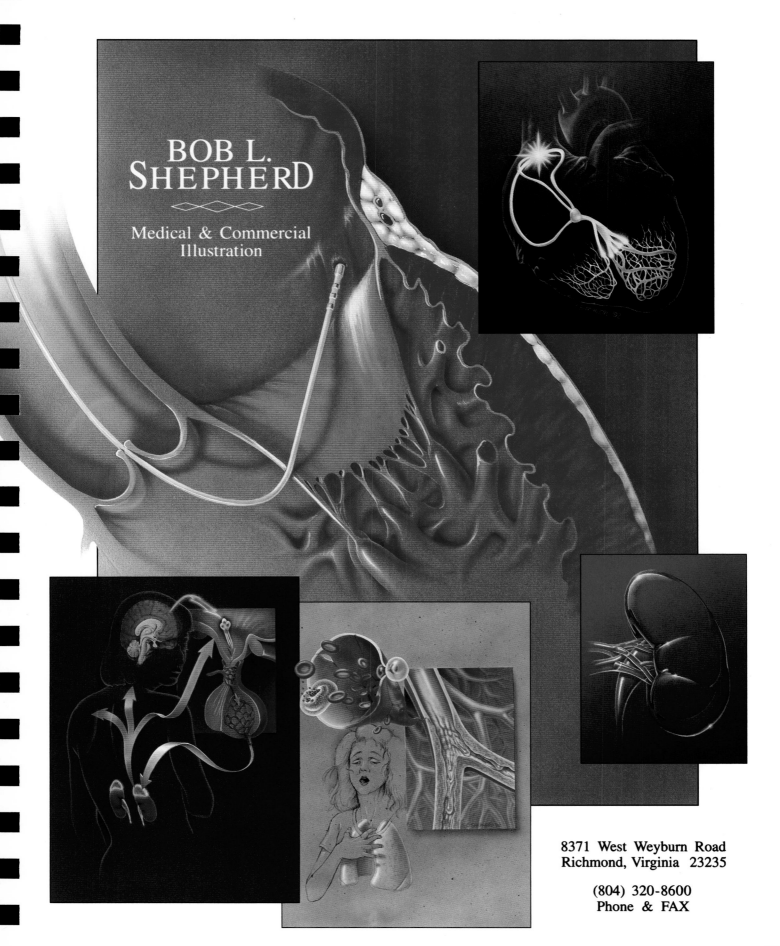

BOB L. SHEPHERD

Medical & Commercial
Illustration

8371 West Weyburn Road
Richmond, Virginia 23235

(804) 320-8600
Phone & FAX

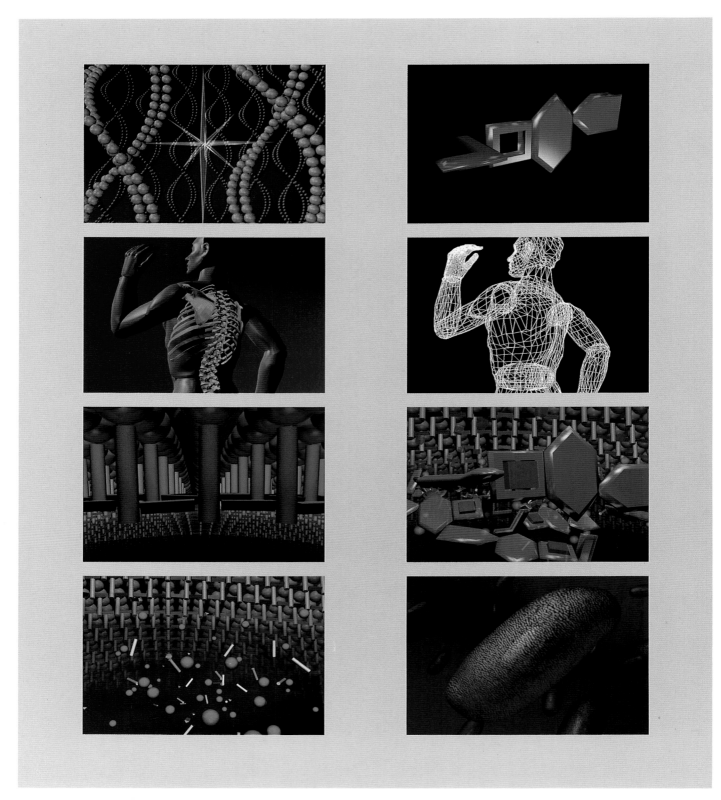

SILICON ARTS, INC.

8305 Route 53 Suite A3
Woodridge, IL 60517
(708) 910-3125
FAX (708) 910-1862

AREAS OF SPECIALIZATION: 3 Dimensional computer graphics and animation for video and print. Special effects/motion for commercial/medical/legal/advertising.

CLIENTS: Leo Burnnet/McDonald's, 3-M, Upjohn, Ameritech, Serta, College of Chiropractics, S.I.U. School of Medicine, and many other corporations, post production facilities, and advertisers.

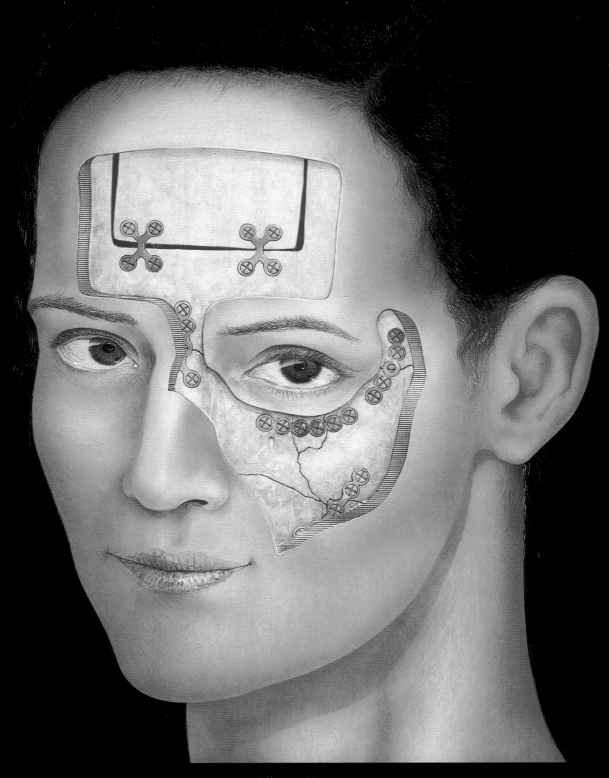

Victor Skersis
Victor Skersis Graphic and Fine Arts
502 Ostrum Street
Bethlehem, PA 18015
(610) 866-5499

NADINE B. SOKOL
221 McDonald Place
St. Louis, Missouri 63119
Tel/Fax: (314) 961-7388

**COMPUTER ART
REFLECTIVE, TONE AND LINE ART**

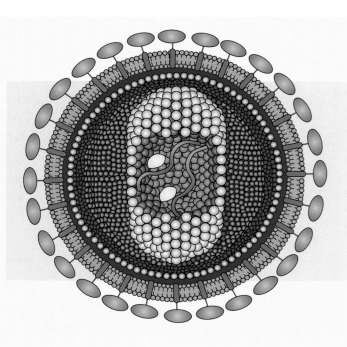

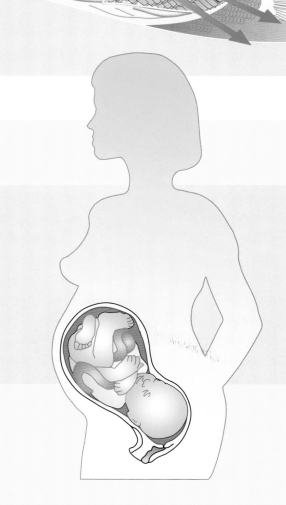

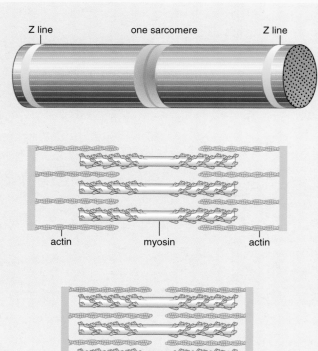

Z line   one sarcomere   Z line

actin   myosin   actin

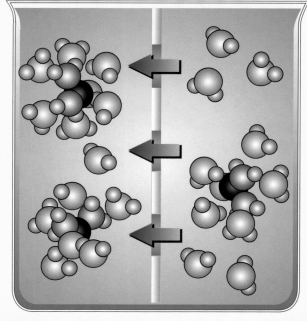

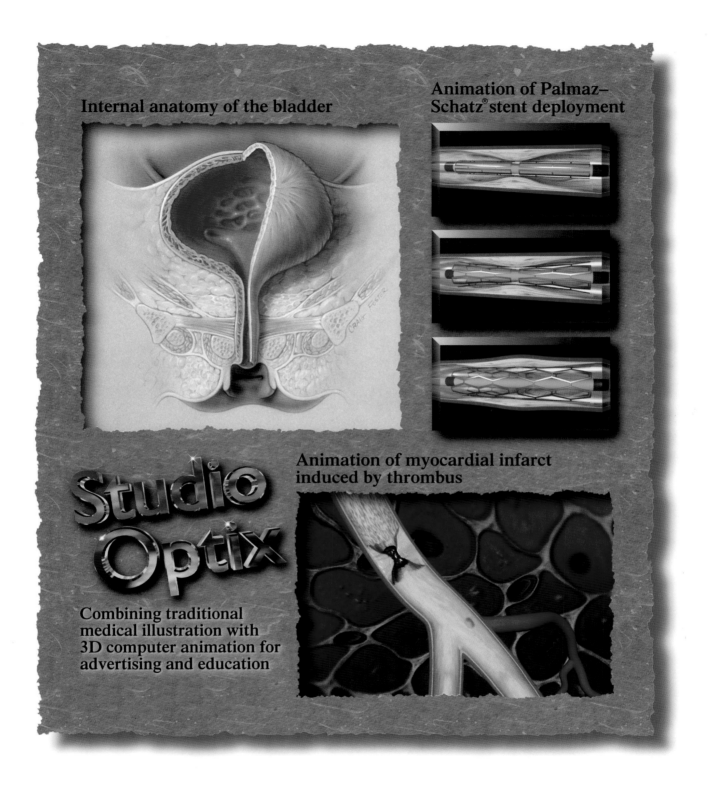

Internal anatomy of the bladder

Animation of Palmaz–Schatz® stent deployment

Animation of myocardial infarct induced by thrombus

Studio Optix

Combining traditional medical illustration with 3D computer animation for advertising and education

STUDIO OPTIX
Craig Foster
103 W. Almeria Road
Phoenix, AZ 85003
(602) 254-4668
FAX (602) 254-7567

AREAS OF SPECIALIZATION: Traditional and computer generated illustration and 3D animation for advertising, editorial, surgical and educational sources. Two years experience with endovascular technologies, cellular, and molecular mechanisms.

CLIENTS: Biotechnology Corporations, Pharmaceutical Companies, Journals, and Private Institutions.

PROFESSIONAL BACKGROUND: University of Michigan School of Art (BFA), Medical College of Georgia (M.S.).

PROFESSIONAL MEMBERSHIPS: Association of Medical Illustrators.

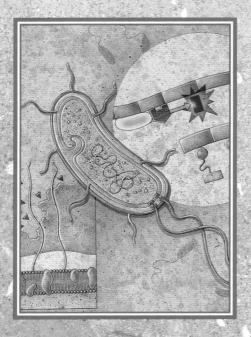

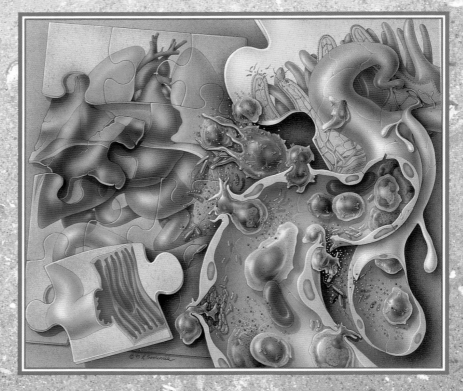

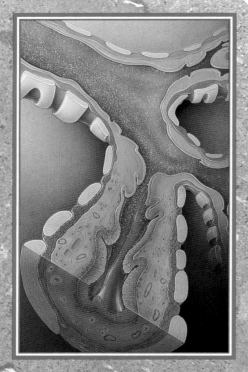

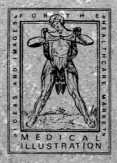

KEVIN A. SOMERVILLE
Medical Illustration

18 Lakeview Street
River Edge, NJ 07661

(201) 488-1026
(201) 488-5867 FAX

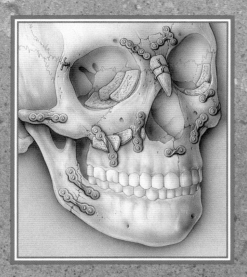

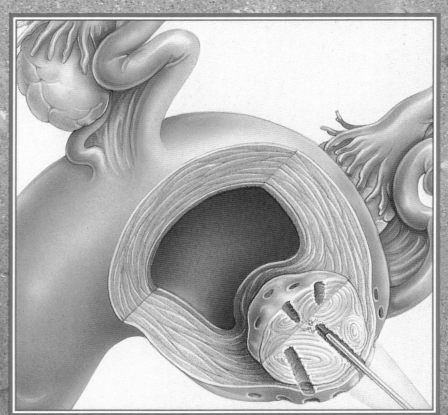

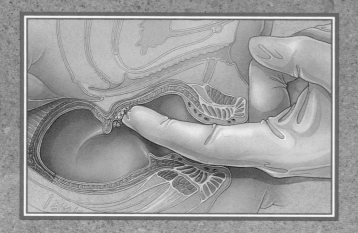

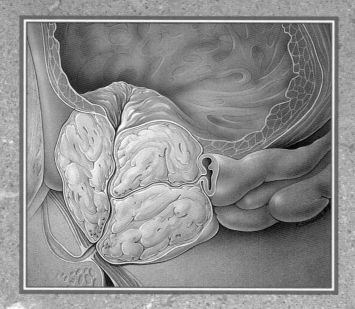

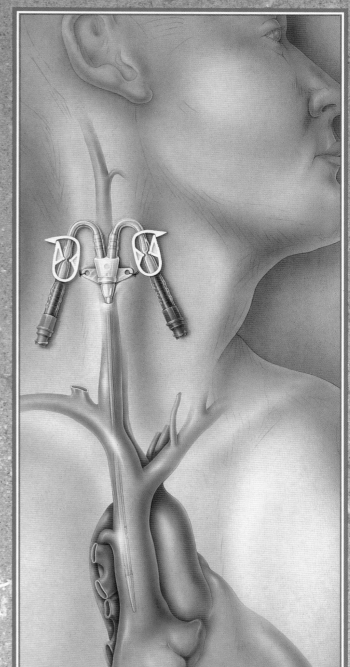

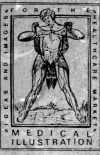

KEVIN A. SOMERVILLE
Medical Illustration

18 Lakeview Street
River Edge, NJ 07661

(201) 488-1026
(201) 488-5867 FAX

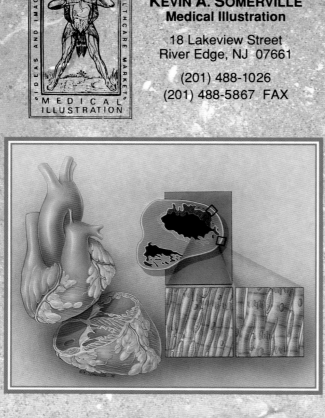

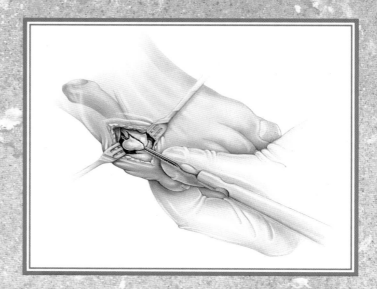

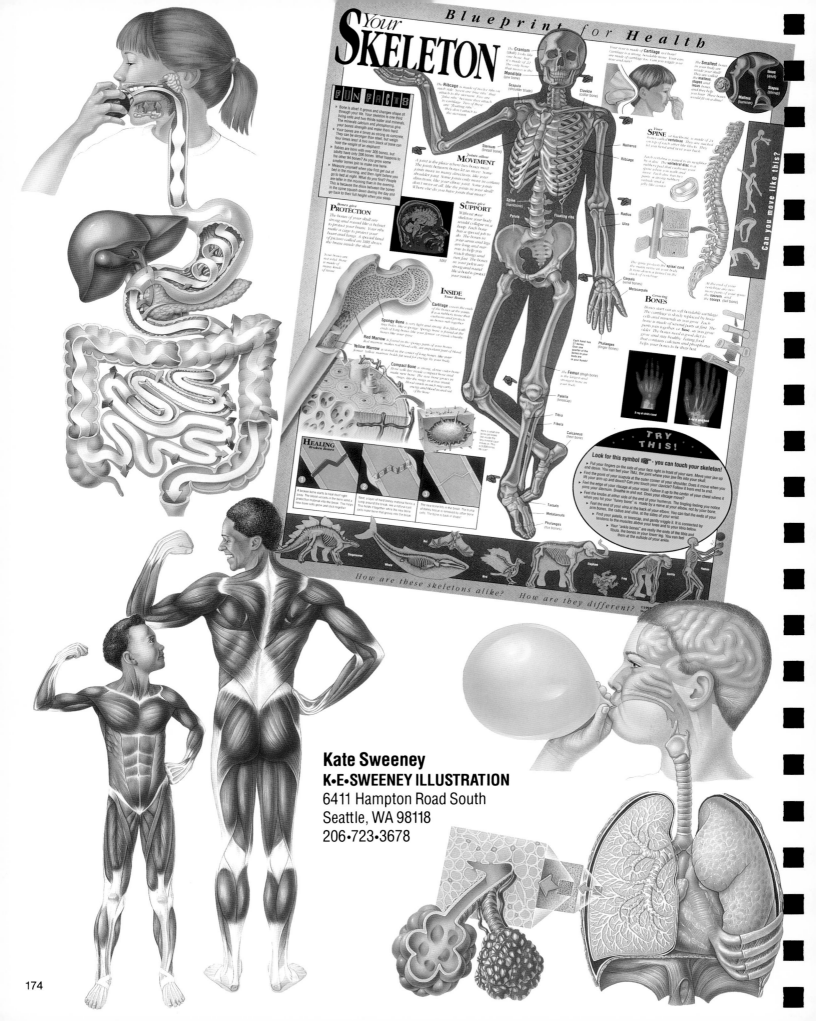

Kate Sweeney
K•E•SWEENEY ILLUSTRATION
6411 Hampton Road South
Seattle, WA 98118
206•723•3678

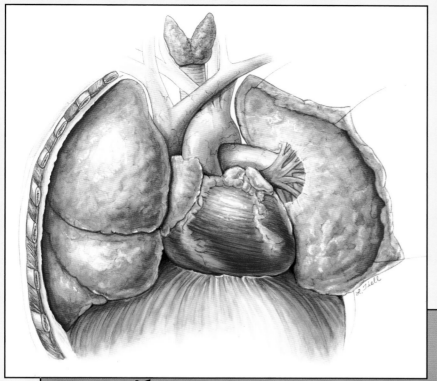

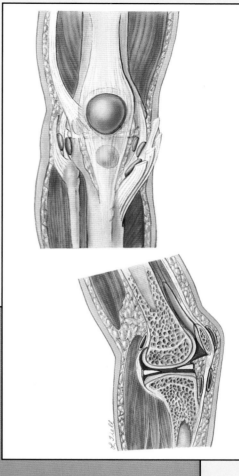

Reptiles

Chapter 5

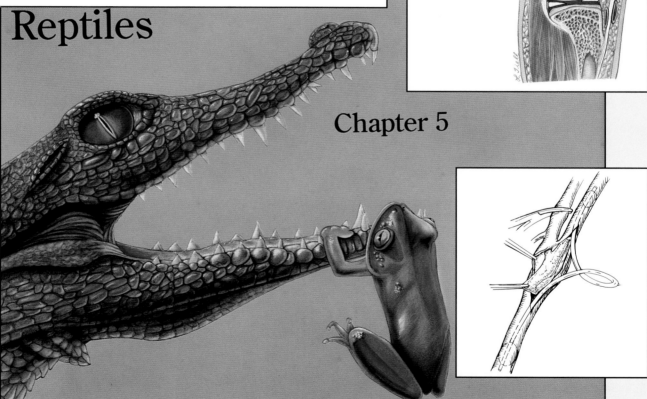

LAURETTA TIELL
88 Richards Road
Columbus, OH 43214
(614) 447-9524

AREAS OF SPECIALIZATION: Anatomical, biological and surgical illustration in full color or black and white. Illustrations for medical and scientific textbooks, patient education materials, advertising and legal presentations.

PROFESSIONAL BACKGROUND: Bachelor of Science, Medical Illustration, Ohio State University.

PROFESSIONAL MEMBERSHIPS: Association of Medical Illustrators.

ELECTRONIC MEDICAL ART

TERRY TOYAMA

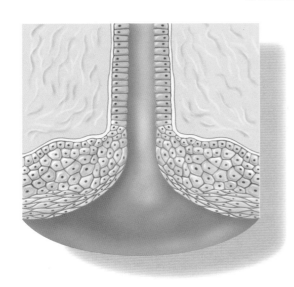

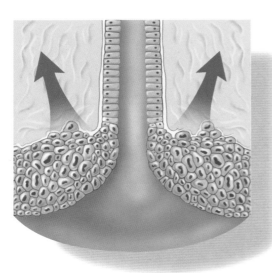

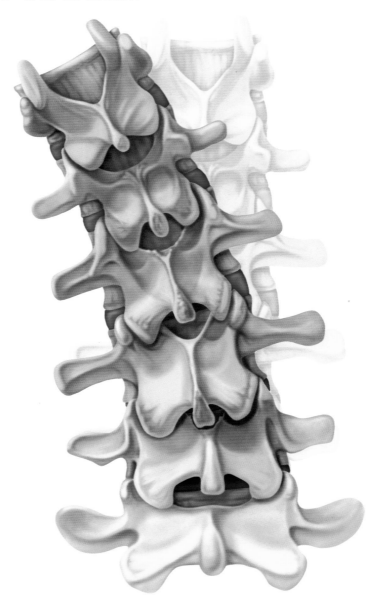

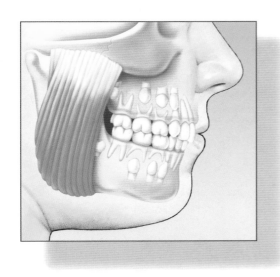

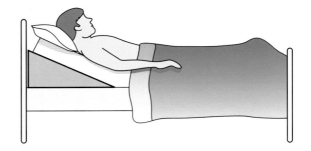

Artwork created using
Adobe Photoshop™ and Illustrator™

60 PARKRIDGE DRIVE, #7 • SAN FRANCISCO, CA 94131 • 415 824 2698

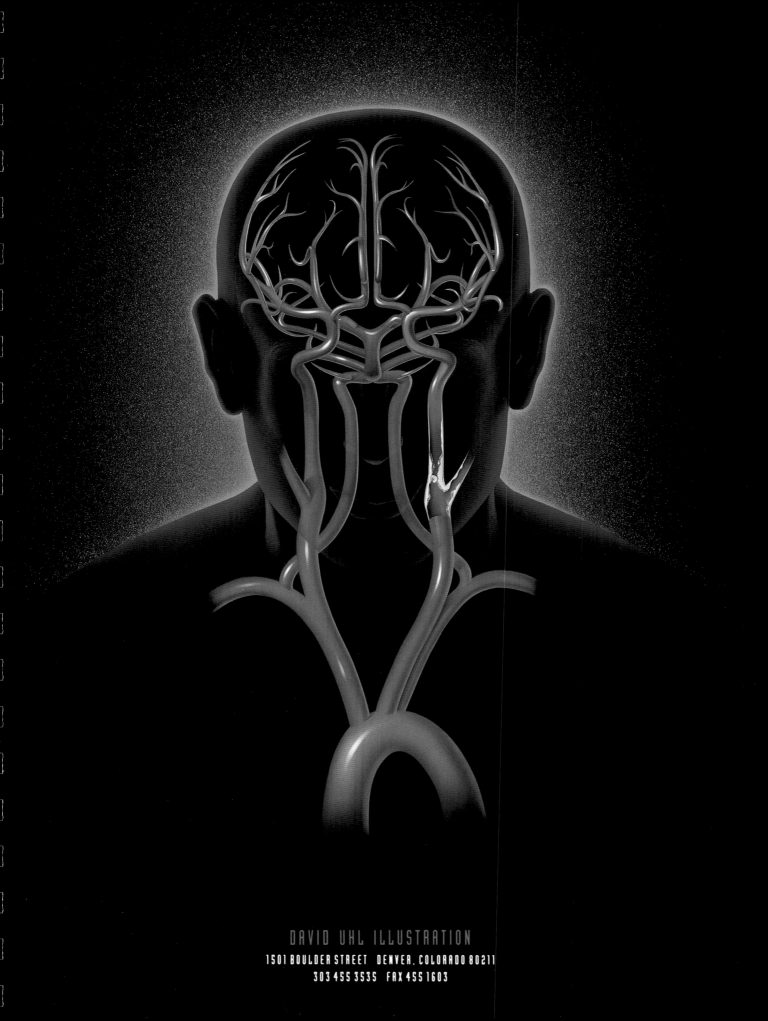

DAVID UHL ILLUSTRATION
1501 BOULDER STREET DENVER, COLORADO 80211
303 455 3535 FAX 455 1603

University of Medicine & Dentistry of New Jersey – Robert Wood Johnson Medical School

MEDIA RESOURCES DEPARTMENT

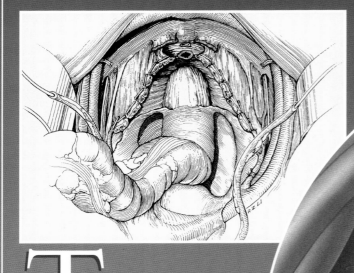

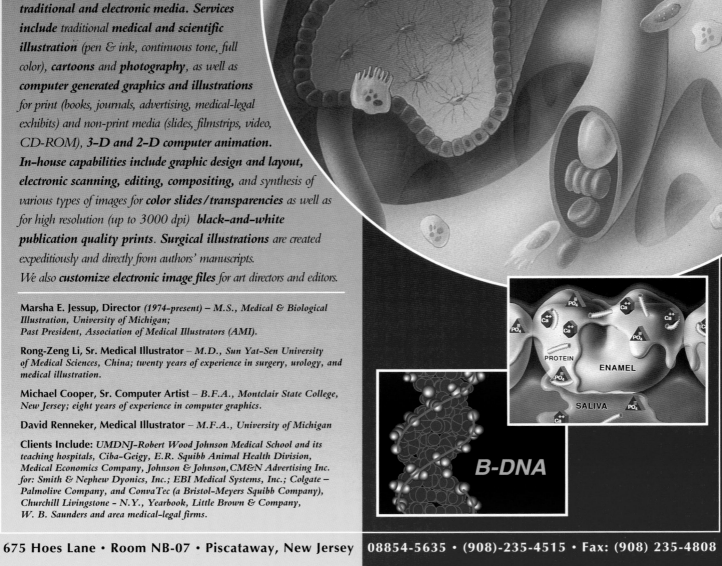

The Department of Media Resources *is a unique blend of talents in* **traditional and electronic media. Services include** *traditional* **medical and scientific illustration** *(pen & ink, continuous tone, full color),* **cartoons** *and* **photography,** *as well as* **computer generated graphics and illustrations** *for print (books, journals, advertising, medical-legal exhibits) and non-print media (slides, filmstrips, video, CD-ROM),* **3-D and 2-D computer animation.** **In-house capabilities include graphic design and layout, electronic scanning, editing, compositing,** *and synthesis of various types of images for* **color slides/transparencies** *as well as for high resolution (up to 3000 dpi)* **black-and-white publication quality prints. Surgical illustrations** *are created expeditiously and directly from authors' manuscripts.*
We also **customize electronic image files** *for art directors and editors.*

Marsha E. Jessup, Director *(1974-present) – M.S., Medical & Biological Illustration, University of Michigan;*
Past President, Association of Medical Illustrators (AMI).

Rong-Zeng Li, Sr. Medical Illustrator *– M.D., Sun Yat-Sen University of Medical Sciences, China; twenty years of experience in surgery, urology, and medical illustration.*

Michael Cooper, Sr. Computer Artist *– B.F.A., Montclair State College, New Jersey; eight years of experience in computer graphics.*

David Renneker, Medical Illustrator *– M.F.A., University of Michigan*

Clients Include: *UMDNJ-Robert Wood Johnson Medical School and its teaching hospitals, Ciba–Geigy, E.R. Squibb Animal Health Division, Medical Economics Company, Johnson & Johnson, CM&N Advertising Inc. for: Smith & Nephew Dyonics, Inc.; EBI Medical Systems, Inc.; Colgate – Palmolive Company, and ConvaTec (a Bristol-Meyers Squibb Company), Churchill Livingstone - N.Y., Yearbook, Little Brown & Company, W. B. Saunders and area medical-legal firms.*

675 Hoes Lane • Room NB-07 • Piscataway, New Jersey 08854-5635 • (908)-235-4515 • Fax: (908) 235-4808

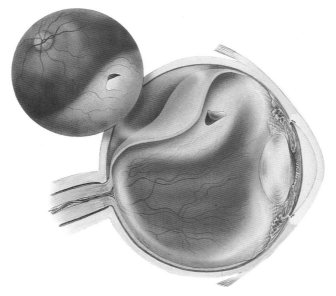

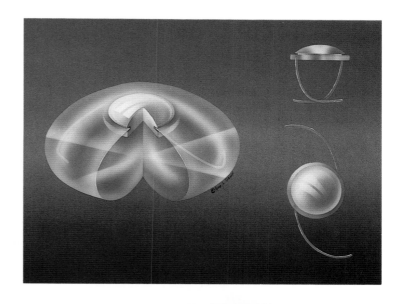

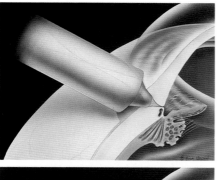

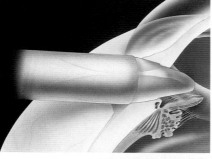

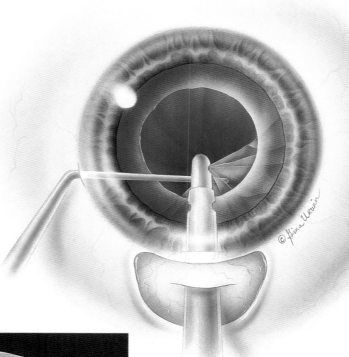

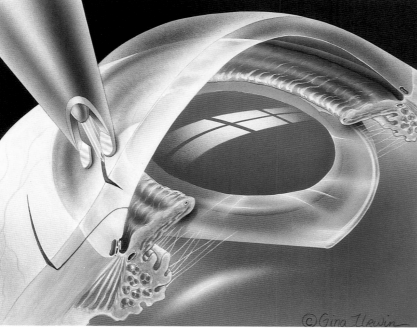

GINA L. URWIN, CMI

Global Illustrations & Design
6418C Reflections Drive
Dublin, Ohio 43017
Phone/Fax (614) 798-8364

Areas of Specialization: *Ophthalmology (normal anatomy, pathology, surgery). Medical and scientific illustrations for textbook, journal and magazine publications, patient education, staff training, slide presentations, promotional brochures.*
Media of expertise: *watercolor and airbrush, pen and ink, various computer graphics programs.*
Professional Membership: *Board Certified Medical Illustrator, The Association of Medical Illustrators.*

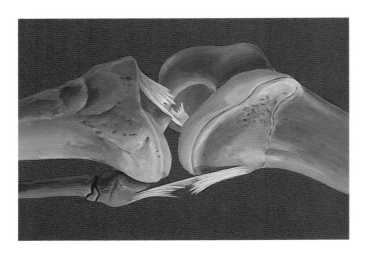

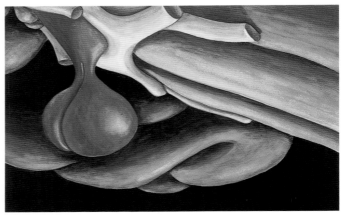

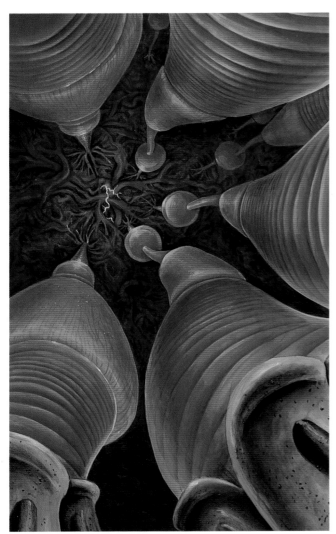

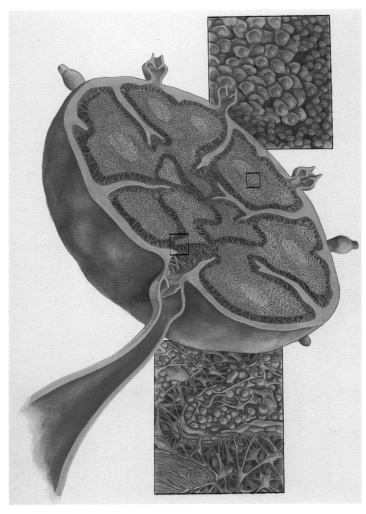

DEAN R. VIGYIKAN
10 Orchard Hill Drive
Orchard Park, NY 14127
(716) 662-5803

AREAS OF SPECIALIZATION: Medical and
Conceptual Illustration

CLIENTS INCLUDE: SLACK Inc. for *Psychi-atric Annals*, Springhouse Corporation for *Nursing '91*, and Laser Graphix of Buffalo, NY.

AWARDS/HONORS: Dean Vigyikan's art has been exhibited in numerous honor shows and received the top medical illustration award at the Rochester Institute of Technology (Rochester, NY). He is noted for his dramatic approach to illustration in color media.

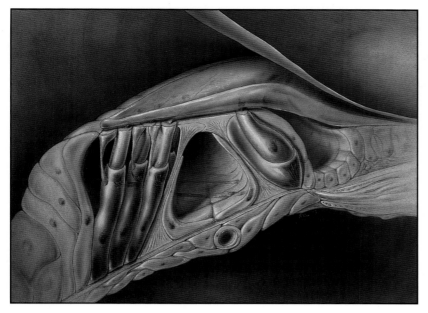

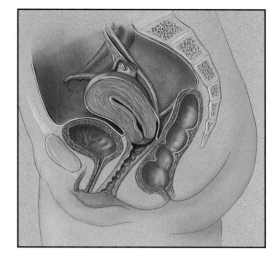

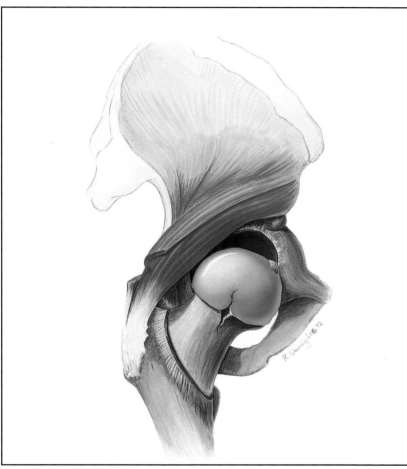

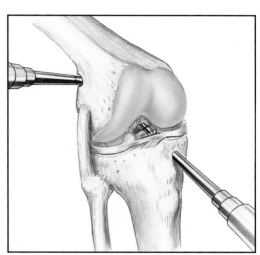

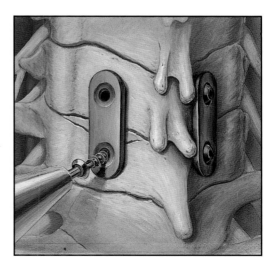

WAINWRIGHT MEDIA, INC.

21 East 22nd Street, Suite 3H
New York, NY 10010
(212) 460-5342
FAX (212) 677-5462

AREAS OF SPECIALIZATION: Computer generated animation and illustration. Traditionally rendered anatomical, surgical, and biological illustration for textbooks, journals and advertising.

PROFESSIONAL BACKGROUND:
Brook Wainwright: B.A., Vassar College; MSMI, Medical College of Georgia.
Robert Wainwright: B.S., Biology, Lehigh University; MSMI, Medical College of Georgia.

PROFESSIONAL MEMBERSHIPS: Association of Medical Illustrators.

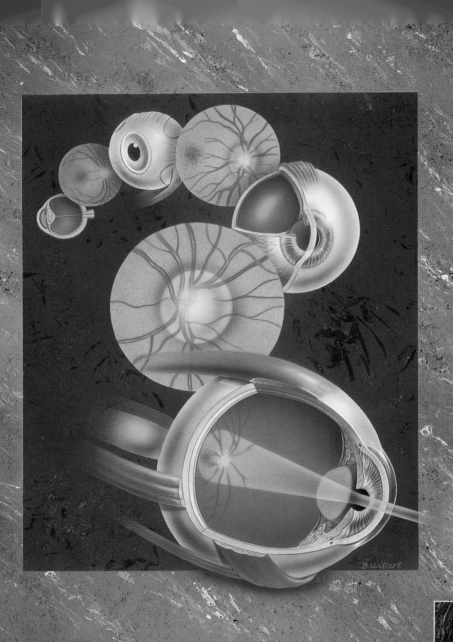

BETH WILLERT
M.S.
MEDICAL
ILLUSTRATOR

4 Woodland Drive, Roselle, NJ 07203

(908) 298-1237 • Fax (908) 298-9148

AREAS OF SPECIALIZATION:
Conceptual, anatomical, surgical
and product illustration in full-color,
continuous tone and line (B&W) for
advertising, editorial, textbook,
exhibition and medical-legal use.

PROFESSIONAL BACKGROUND:
B.A., Art, and B.S. Biology, Michigan
State University. M.S., Medical and
Biological Illustration, University of
Michigan . Two-year staff position,
Children's Hospital National Medical
Center in Washington, D.C. Freelance
since 1982. Board Certified.

PROFESSIONAL MEMBERSHIPS:
Association of Medical Illustrators,
Graphic Artists Guild (1983-1993),
Guild of Natural Science Illustrators,
Society of Illustrators-New York.

© B. Willert 1994

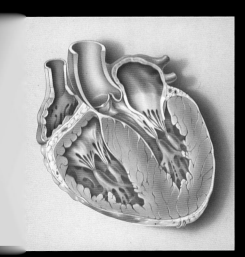

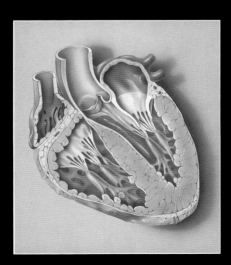

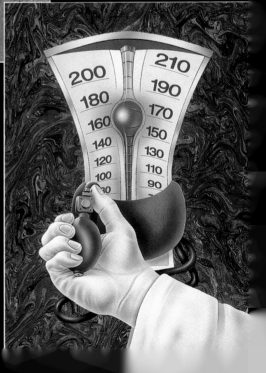

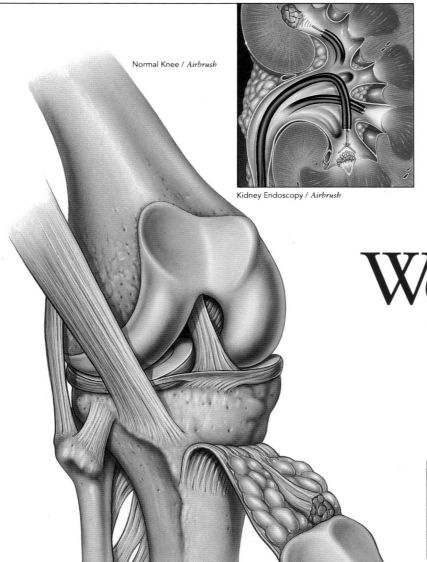

Normal Knee / *Airbrush*

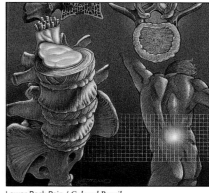

Kidney Endoscopy / *Airbrush*

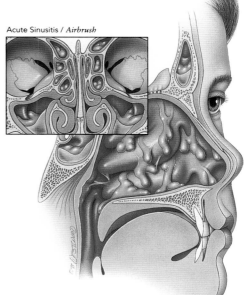

Lower Back Pain / *Colored Pencil*

Westwood

William B. Westwood, MS

915 Broadway, Albany, New York 12207
Phone: (518) 432-5237
Fax: (518) 432-7106

Acute Sinusitis / *Airbrush*

- Over 22 years experience, including 10 years as a surgical illustrator at the **Mayo Clinic**, serving clients nationally.

- **Board certified**, broadly experienced in all areas of anatomy and surgery with special expertise in ENT, gynecology, orthopedics, as well as the cardiovascular and immune systems.

- Over 30 awards for **creative excellence**.

- Conceptual and anatomic medical art for journal ads, posters, patient education, product promotion and video.

Chronic Renal Failure / *Airbrush*

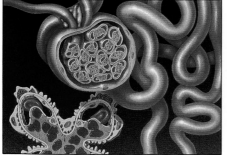

Cervical Spondylosis / *Colored Pencil*

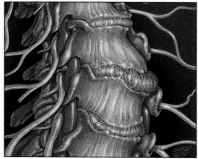

Virus Induced Asthma / *Airbrush*

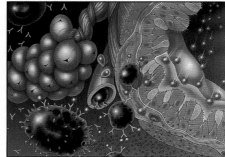

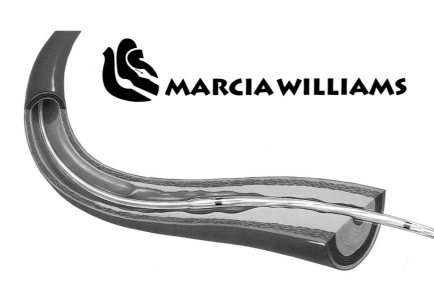

MARCIA WILLIAMS

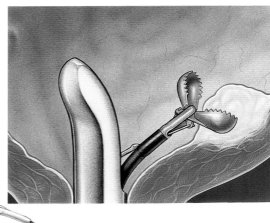

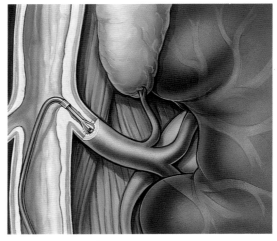

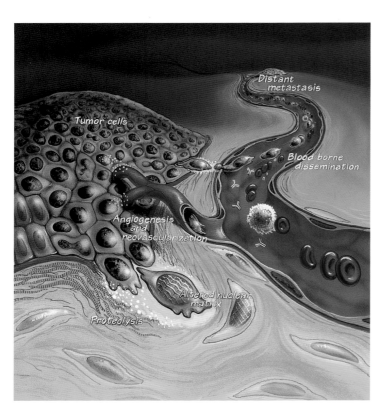

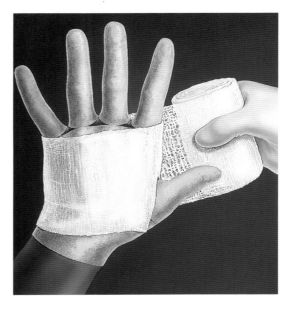

MARCIA WILLIAMS
84 Duncklee Street
Newton Highlands, MA 02161
(617) 558-1092

Medical product illustration, as well as surgical and anatomical illustration in color, tone and line. Extensive knowledge of medical and surgical procedures based on over 15 years of working with physicians, surgeons, nurses and scientists.

Master's degree in medical illustration. Free-lance since 1983. Formerly medical illustrator at Boston University Medical Center. Please call for samples of line illustrations.

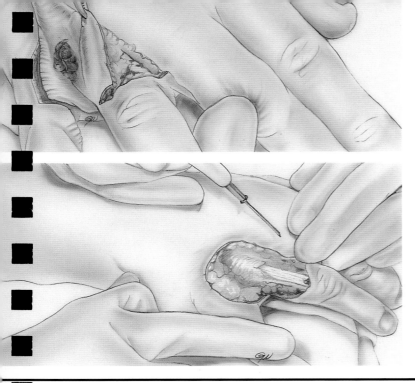

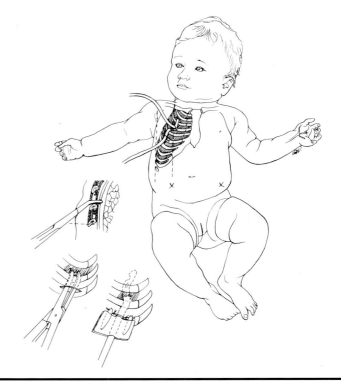

WILSON WILSON
Illustration & Communication Inc.

GENEVIEVE M. WILSON
GERALD D. WILSON
22 El Mirador
Nicasio, California 94946
(415) 662-2040
FAX (415) 662-2408

PROFESSIONAL BACKGROUND:
Genevieve Wilson: B.F.A., California College of Arts and Crafts, M.A., Medical Illustration, University of Texas.
Gerald D. Wilson: B.A., Stanford University, Graphic Design; Landor Associates; Primo Angeli Graphics, San Francisco.
PROFESSIONAL MEMBERSHIPS:
AFA, AMI, DESA, GNSI, California State Coroners Association, International Association of Identification.

AREAS OF SPECIALIZATION:
Conceptual, educational and instructional biomedical illustration. Line, tone and full color. Specializing in anatomical, surgical, and forensic applications for textbooks, medical and pharmaceutical publications, advertising, editorial and cover art. Medical legal and veterinary illustration.
OTHER: Composite police art, facial aging, skull reconstruction.

CLIENTS: AAHA, ad agencies, Appleton Lange, BioGrowth, Inc., Compendium for Veterinarians, District Attorneys, Hanley & Belfus, HBJ, hospitals, Hospital Practice, law firms, Lawrence Berkeley Lab, Lions Eye Bank, Lippincott, McGraw-Hill, Oxford University Press, Primary Cardiology, Raven Press, Raychem Corporation, Stuart Pharmaceutical, Syntex, Thieme, UC Berkeley, U.S. Park Service, Williams & Wilkins.

Arthroplasty of the Shoulder

Richard J. Friedman

Thieme

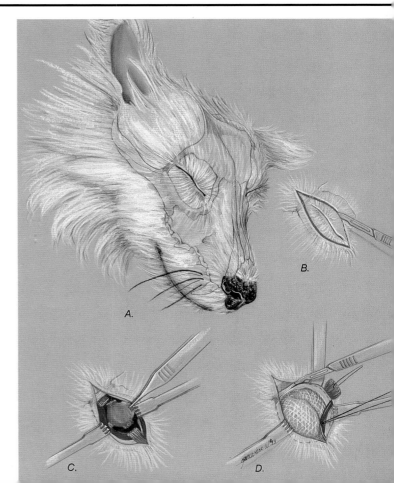

A.

B.

C.

D.

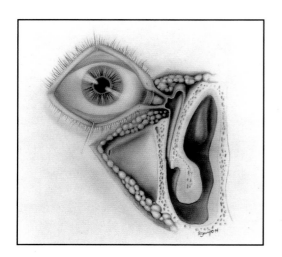

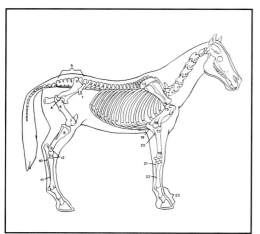

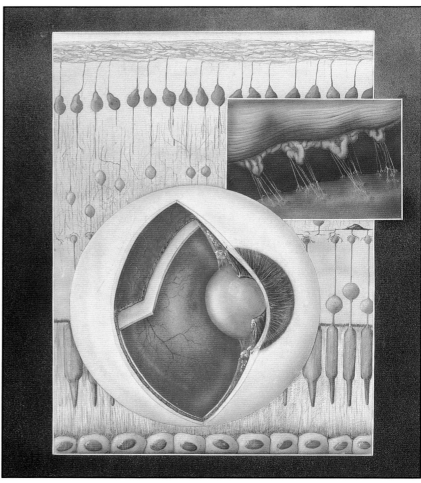

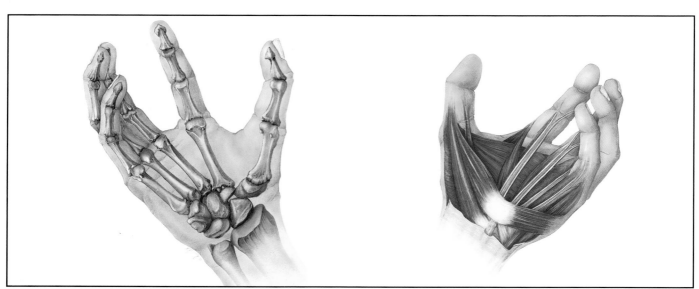

BETH A. YOUNG
6469 Rt. 86
Windsor, OH 44099
(216) 272-5453

AREAS OF SPECIALIZATION: Colour, half-tone and pen & ink illustrations. Anatomical, biological and surgical topics for use in advertising, textbooks and periodicals, as well as legal and educational presentations.

CLIENTS: Client list available upon request.

PROFESSIONAL BACKGROUND: B.F.A., Medical Illustration, Cleveland Institute of Art; Case Western Reserve School of Medicine.

PROFESSIONAL MEMBERSHIPS: Association of Medical Illustrators, Guild of Natural Science Illustrators.

Medical Sculptures and Working Models for Print, Exhibition and Film

Mark Yurkiw & Company make working models and three dimensional illustrations that speak directly and accurately to scientists, physicians and laymen alike. They supply accurate sculptural illustrations to clients including Squibb, Merck, Pfizer, CIBA-GEIGY, Warner Lambert and Osteonics.

The company's artistic team has an extensive background in science, medicine, and sculpture. An integral part of that team is Caspar Henselmann, veteran medical model maker and a longtime member of the Association of Medical Illustrators. Geared toward problem solving, they work in a facility fully equipped for research, development and fabrication. Yurkiw models have decisively demonstrated implants, joint replacements, other medical procedures as well as the effects of drugs. Technical accuracy and precision are a promise.

Background:
Model and Effects:
Testosterone Patch;
Client: Alza;
Photographer:
David Wagner

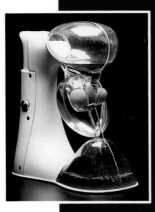

Left:
Model: Working Prostate;
Client: Merck;
Photographer:
James Kozyra

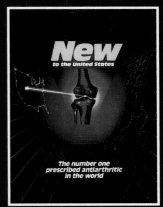

Above:
Model: Transparent Bones and Map;
Client: CIBA-GEIGY;
Photographer:
Carmen Macedonia

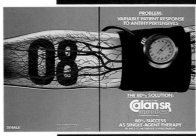

Above:
Model: Transparent Arm and Sphygmo-manometer;
Client: Searle;
Art Director:
Len Obsatz

MARK YURKIW AND CO.

MY!

MODELMAKERS/SPECIAL EFFECTS

MARK YURKIW AND COMPANY
180 VARICK STREET N.Y., NY 10014
212-229-0741 FAX 229-0734

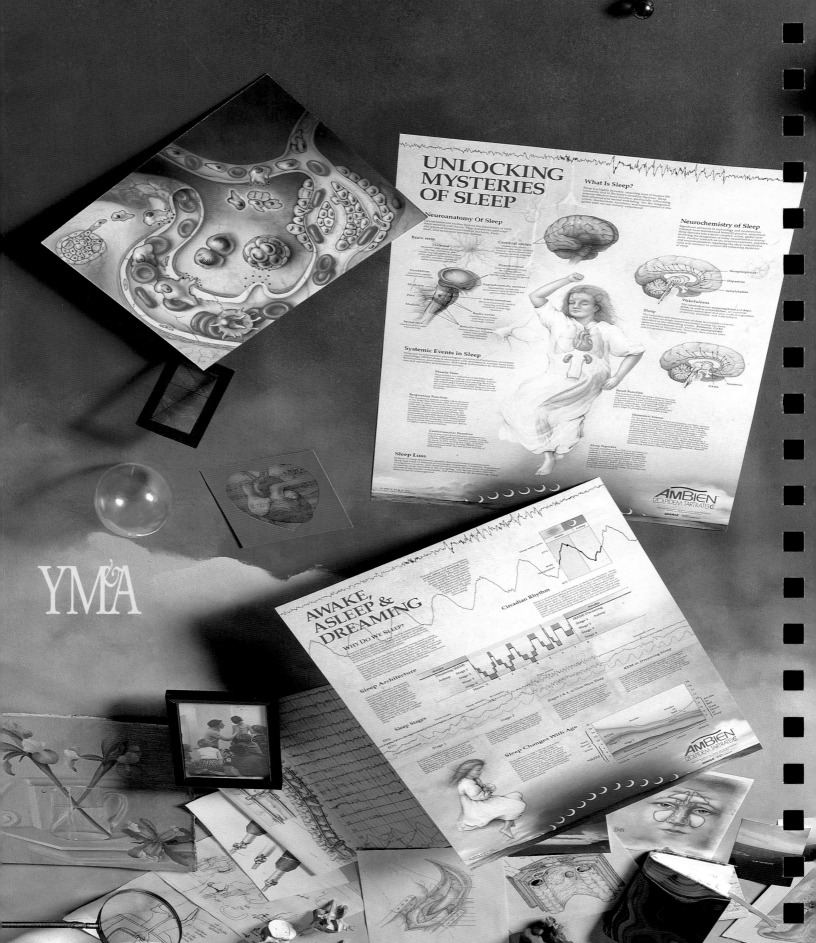

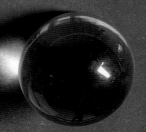

CHRISTINE D. YOUNG

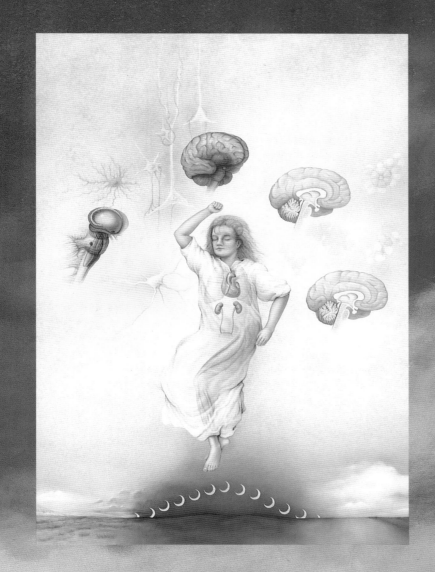

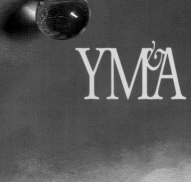

YM&A

YOUNG, MCKENNA & ASSOCIATES, INC.

Art
for
Science,
Health
and
Medicine

2106 Maple Avenue
Evanston, IL
60201-2702
Voice 708.866.9388
Fax 708.866.9390

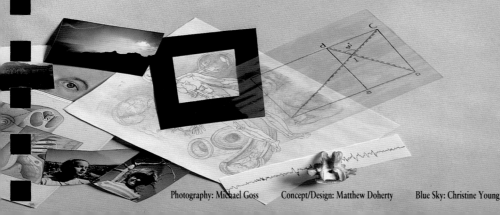

Photography: Michael Goss   Concept/Design: Matthew Doherty   Blue Sky: Christine Young   ©1994 YM&A, Inc.

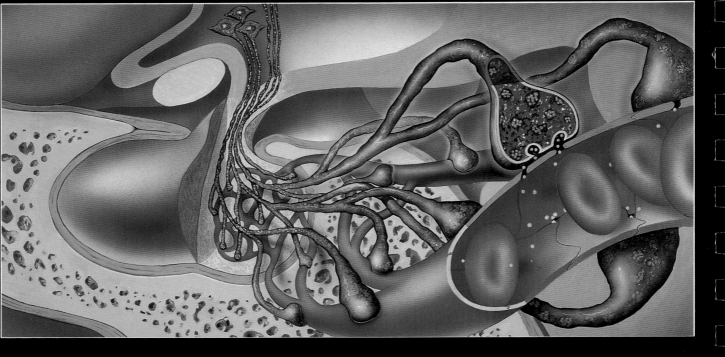

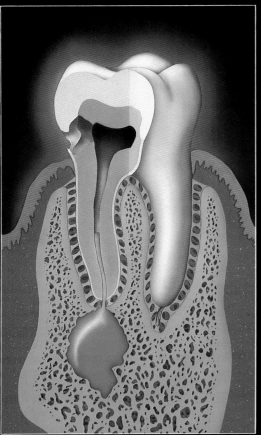

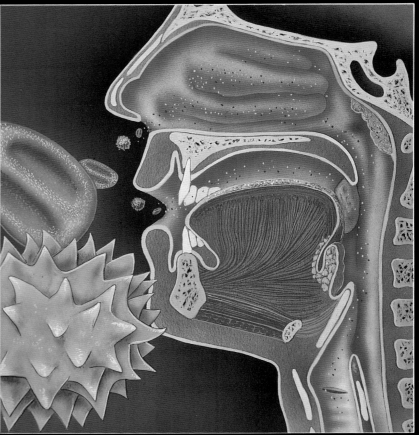

E D   Z I L B E R T S

SPECIALIZING IN CONCEPTUAL MEDICAL & ANATOMICAL ILLUSTRATIONS OF THE HEAD AND NECK
FOR ADVERTISING, PUBLISHING, AND CORPORATE HEALTH CARE COMPANIES

5690 DTC Blvd. #190 • Englewood, CO 80111 • **TEL: (303) 220-5040** • FAX: (303) 770-8509

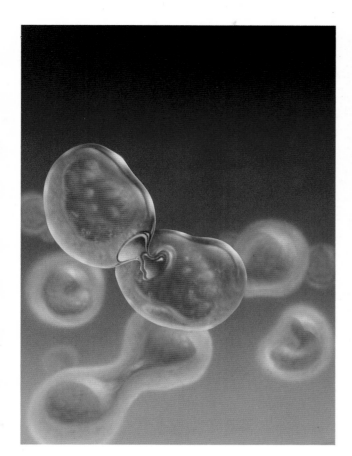

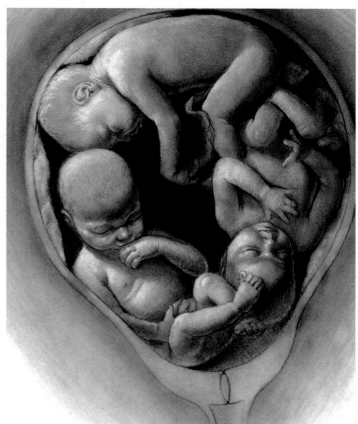

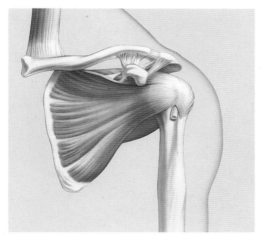

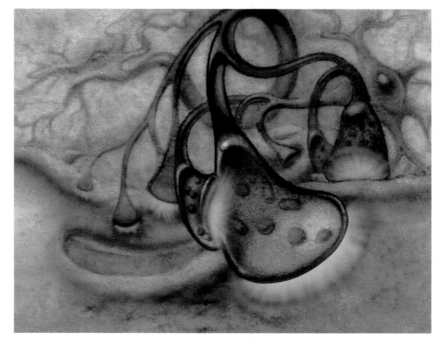

CRAIG ZUCKERMAN
109 Carthage Road
Scarsdale, NY 10583
(914) 725-6004
FAX (212) 924-8683